DSM-5 Insanely Simplified

DSM-5 INSANELY SIMPLIFIED

Unlocking the Spectrums within DSM-5 and ICD 10

Steven Buser, MD
&
Leonard Cruz, MD

Illustrations by Luke Sloan

innerQuest
Asheville, North Carolina

www.ChironPublicatons.com
innerQuest is a book imprint of Chiron Publications

Cover design by Cornelia G. Murariu

Printed in the United States of America

ISBN 978-1-63051-207-1   paperback
ISBN 978-1-63051-208-8   clothbound
ISBN 978-1-63051-209-5   electronic

Library of Congress Cataloging-in-Publication Data

Buser, Steven, 1963- , author.
 DSM-5 insanely simplified : unlocking the spectrums within DSM-5 & ICD 10 / Steven Buser, Leonard Cruz.
    p. ; cm.
 Includes bibliographical references and index.
 ISBN 978-1-63051-207-1 (pbk. : alk. paper) -- ISBN 978-1-63051-208-8 (clothbound : alk. paper) -- ISBN 978-1-63051-209-5 (electronic)
 I. Cruz, Leonard, 1957- , author. II. Title.
 [DNLM: 1. Diagnostic and statistical manual of mental disorders. 5th ed. 2. International statistical classification of diseases and related health problems. 10th revision. 3. Mental Disorders--classification--Handbooks. 4. Mental Disorders--diagnosis--Handbooks. WM 34]

 RC455.2.C4
 616.89'075--dc23

2014041424

To our wives, Megan and Vicky, and our children,
Brian, Emily, Saila and Sarah
And all their amazing love and inspiration
that fuel our life's work.

CONTENTS

DSM-5 SUMMARY PAGES

WARNING! The description of DSM-5 disorders that follows are in a highly simplified and summarized form. They are meant to give a quick overview and a reminder of the disorder. They do not, however, include all of the full diagnostic criterion found in the complete DSM-5 text. The DSM-5 should be purchased as a separate side-by-side text. Please do not use this book to formally reach a diagnosis, but rather as a quick reference and memory tool.

All codes begin with DSM-5 and following the backslash include the ICD-10 codes (most of which begin with a "F")

DEPRESSIVE DISORDERS
Major Depressive Disorder
- 5 "SIG E CAPSS" symptoms for at least 2 weeks [Sadness, Interest loss, Guilt or worthlessness, Energy loss, Concentration loss, Appetite change, Psychomotor agitation or retardation, Sleep change, Suicidal thoughts]

296.2x / F32.x   Major Depressive Disorder, single episode
296.3x / F33.x   Major Depressive Disorder, recurrent

Intensity:	Single Episode:	Recurrent Episode:
Mild	296.21 / F32.0	296.31 / F33.0
Moderate	296.22 / F32.1	296.32 / F33.1
Severe	296.23 / F32.2	296.33 / F33.2
Psychotic	296.24 / F32.3	296.34 / F33.3

300.4 / F34.1 Persistent Depressive Disorder (Dysthymia)
- Sad most days for 2 years
- 2 or more of: sleep change, hopelessness, appetite change, low self-esteem, concentration loss
- Never 2 months symptom free in first 2 years
- Significant distress or impairment

296.99 / F34.8 Disruptive Mood Dysregulation Disorder
- Severe recurrent temper outbursts (verbal or physical)
- Out of proportion to context
- 3 or more per week; persists more than a year; began as child (6-18)
- Persistent irritability
- (not better explained by mania, depression, autism, substance abuse, etc)

625.4 / N94.3 Premenstrual Dysphoric Disorder
- Symptoms present one week prior to menses
- At least 1 of the 4 following: mood swings, irritability/anger, sadness, anxiety/tension
- At least 5 total: mood swings, irritability/anger, sadness, anxiety/tension, loss of interest, poor concentration, fatigue, appetite change, sleep change, overwhelmed, physical symptoms (breast tenderness, bloating, pain, weight gain)
- Significant distress or impairment

BIPOLAR DISORDERS
296.7 / F31.9 Bipolar I Disorder
- Euphoric or irritable mood and increased energy or activity for 1 week
- 3 out of 7: grandiose, decreased sleep, talkative, racing thoughts, distractibility, increased goal-directed activity, impulsive
- Social or work impairment

296.89 / F31.81 Bipolar II Disorder
- At least 1 Hypomanic episode and at least 1 Major Depressive episode
- No full Manic episodes

Hypomanic Episode:
- Same as Bipolar I Manic episode except: at least 4 days duration (instead of 7)
- And **NO marked impairment** in social or occupational functioning

301.13 / F34.0 Cyclothymic Disorder
- Numerous hypomania and depression symptoms for most of the time for 2 years
- Never reaches full diagnosis for either hypomanic, manic or depressive episodes
- Not without symptoms for 2 months in 1st 2 years.
- Clinically significant distress or impairment

May Add Specifiers:
with Anxious Distress
with Mixed Features (mania and depression)
with Rapid Cycling (for Bipolar I and II: > 4 episodes per year)
with Melancholic Features (loss of pleasure, lack of reactivity, despair, worse in a.m., early morning awakening)
with Atypical Features (weight gain, increased sleep, leaden paralysis, interpersonal rejection sensitivity, mood reactivity)
with Psychotic Features, with Catatonia, with Peripartum Onset, with Seasonal Pattern

PSYCHOTIC DISORDERS
295.90 / F20.9 Schizophrenia
- Must have 1 positive symptom (hallucinations, delusions or disorganized speech) for 1 month
- 2 of the following: hallucinations, delusions, disorganized speech, disorganized behavior, or negative symptoms (low emotion, low motivation)
- Prior or residual poor functioning for at least 6 months
- Social or work impairment

295.40 / F20.81 Schizophreniform Disorder
- Schizophrenic symptoms between 1-6 months duration

295.70 / F25.0 Schizoaffective Disorder, Bipolar type
- Schizophrenic symptoms and Bipolar I symptoms present most of the time
- At least 2 weeks of delusions or hallucinations without Bipolar symptoms
- Must have Bipolar symptoms for the majority of time.

295.70 / F25.1 Schizoaffective Disorder, Depressive type
- Schizophrenic symptoms and Depression symptoms present most of the time.
- At least 2 weeks of delusions or hallucinations without Depression symptoms
- Must have Depression symptoms for the majority of time

297.1 / F22 Delusional Disorder
- Moderate delusions at least 1 month, not Schizophrenic level
- Otherwise good functioning; no bizarre behavior
  - Erotomanic type
  - Grandiose type
  - Jealous type
  - Persecutory type
  - Somatic type
  - Mixed type
  - Unspecified type

298.8 / F23 Brief Psychotic Disorder
- Schizophrenic symptoms for less than 1 month
- Full return to premorbid level
  - with marked stressors
  - without marked stressors
  - with postpartum onset
  - with Catatonia

ANXIETY DISORDERS
300.01 / F41.0 Panic Disorder
- Recurrent, abrupt, unexpected intense fear or discomfort
- Persistent worry of additional attacks for 1 month
- 4 out of 13 symptoms: (palpitations, sweating, trembling, shortness of breath, choking, chest pain, nausea, dizziness, derealization, fear of "going crazy", fear of dying, numbness/ tingling, hot/cold flashes)
- "Panic Attack" can also be a specifier for other diagnoses (i.e. "PTSD with Panic Attacks")

300.22 / F40.00 Agoraphobia
- Intense fear of 2 or more of: public transportation, open spaces (markets, bridges), enclosed spaced (theaters, shops), crowds, being away from home
- Avoids these areas
- Greater than 6 months; interferes with work or social functioning

300.02 / F41.1 Generalized Anxiety Disorder
- Excessive worry most days for 6 months
- 3 out of 6: (restless, fatigue, decreased concentration, irritability, tense, insomnia)
- Interferes with work / social functioning

300.29 Specific Phobia
- Intense unreasonable fear
- Interferes with work / social functioning

F40.218 - Animal fear (insects, snakes, dogs, etc)
F40.228 - Natural environment (heights, thunderstorms, etc)
F40.230 - Blood
F40.231 - Needle injections
F40.232 - Other medical fears
F40.233 - Fear of injury
F40.248 - Situational (elevators, planes, tight spaces)
F40.298 - Other

300.23 / F40.10 Social Anxiety Disorder
- Formerly "Social Phobia"
- Persistent fear of social interaction or performance
- Interferes with work / social functioning

309.21 / F93.0 Separation Anxiety Disorder
- Excessive anxiety over separation from home or parents

312.23 / F94.0 Selective Mutism
- Mute in some settings but not others

OBSESSIVE-COMPULSIVE DISORDERS
300.3 / F42 Obsessive-Compulsive Disorder
- Obsessions: persistent intrusive, inappropriate non-psychotic thoughts
- Compulsions: repetitive behaviors compelled to reduce distress
- Patient sees as excessive / unreasonable
- Marked distress / interference

300.7 / F45.22 Body Dysmorphic Disorder
- Preoccupation with imagined defect in physical appearance
- Repetitive checking, grooming, picking, comparing, or reassurance seeking
- Work / social impairment

312.39 / F63.2 Trichotillomania
- Recurrent hair pulling and hair loss
- Failed attempts to stop hair pulling
- Marked distress or impairment

300.3 / F42 Hoarding Disorder
- Can't discard possessions regardless of value
- Possessions accumulate, cluttering living space
- Marked distress or impairment

698.4 / L98.1 Excoriation (Skin-Picking) Disorder
- Persistent skin picking causing lesions or infections
- Failed attempts to stop skin picking
- Marked distress or impairment

SUBSTANCE ABUSE DISORDERS
Alcohol Use Disorder
305.00 / F10.10 MILD=2-3 symptoms
303.90 / F10.20 MOD = 4-5 symptoms
303.90 / F10.20 SEV = 6 or more symptoms

Symptom List:

- Uses more than intended
- Failed attempts to cut back
- Excessive time spent in obtaining, using, or recovering from substance
- Cravings for substance
- Substance use leads to problems at work, school or home
- Important work, social or recreational activities are given up due to substance use
- Uses in dangerous situations
- Persistent use despite awareness of problem
- Tolerance (needs more substance for same effect)
- Withdrawals

Alcohol Use, Intoxication, or Withdrawal Disorders
Caffeine Intoxication or Withdrawal Disorders
Cannabis Use, Intoxication, or Withdrawal Disorders
Hallucinogen Use or Intoxication Disorders
Inhalant Use or Intoxication Disorders
Opioid Use, Intoxication, or Withdrawal Disorders
Sedative Use, Intoxication, or Withdrawal Disorders
Stimulant (Cocaine / Amphetamine) Use, Intoxication, or Withdrawal Disorders
Tobacco Use or Withdrawal Disorders

312.31 / F63.0 Gambling Disorder
- Continued gambling despite distress or impairment
- 4 of the following: increasing amounts of money gambled, irritable when cuts back on gambling, failed attempts to cut back, preoccupied with gambling, gambles to feel better, "chases their losses" (gambles later to make their money back), lies about gambling, relationship / work / or school problems, others give them money to help desperate need caused by losses

NEURODEVELOPMENTAL DISORDERS
Attention-Deficit / Hyperactivity Disorder (ADHD)
- Persistent **inattention** or **hyperactivity** interfering with functioning for 6 months, began before age of 12
- **Inattention**- 6 or more of the following: inattention to details, difficulty sustaining attention, doesn't listen well, poor follow through on tasks, poor organization, avoids homework or large projects, often loses things, distractible, forgetful
- **Hyperactivity** - 6 or more of the following: fidgets or squirms, leaves seat often, runs around inappropriately, can't play quietly, driven, always moving, overly talkative, blurts out answers, difficulty waiting or taking turns, interrupts frequently

314.01 / F90.2 ADHD, Combined
314.00 / F90.0 ADHD, Inattentive
314.01 / F90.1 ADHD, Hyperactive / Impulsive

299.00 / F84.0 Autism Spectrum Disorder:
Problems with social communication and social interaction
Repetitive behaviors; 2 of the following:
- Repetitive actions or speech
- Insistence on sameness
- Restricted fixated interests
- Increased or decreased sensitivity to sensory stimulation
3 Levels:
Level 1 - requiring support
Level 2 - requiring substantial support
Level 3 - requiring very substantial support

Communication Disorders:
315.39 / F80.9 Language Disorder - difficulty using language
315.39 / F80.0 Speech Sound Disorder - difficulty speaking
315.35 / F80.81 Childhood Onset Fluency Disorder - stuttering issues
315.39 / F80.89 Social (Pragmatic) Communication Disorder - speaking difficulties in social context

Specific Learning Disorders:
315.00 / F81.0 Learning Disorder in Reading
315.2 / F81.81 Learning Disorder in Writing
315.1 / F81.2 Learning Disorder in Mathematics

319 Intellectual Disability [F70 - Mild; F71 - Moderate; F72 - Severe; F73 - Profound]
- Decreased intellectual functioning
- Decreased developmental and social functioning
- Begins in childhood

Motor Disorders:
315.4 / F82 Developmental Coordination Disorder
- Coordination impairment, clumsy, slow, inaccurate
- Marked distress / interference

307.3 / F98.4 Stereotypic movement Disorder
- Repetitive purposeless movement (head banging, rocking, biting, picking, hitting, etc.)
- Interferes with functioning or self-injurious

307.23 / F95.2 Tourette's Disorder
- Multiple motor tics + 1 vocal tic
- Persistent for 1 year
- Marked distress or impairment
- Onset before 18 years old

307.22 / F95.1 Persistent Motor or Vocal Tic Disorder
- Motor only or vocal only tics
- Persistent for 1 year
- Marked distress or impairment
- Onset before 18 years old

307.21 / F95.0 Provisional Tic Disorder
- Tics, 4 weeks to 1 year
- Marked distress or impairment
- Onset before 18 years old

TRAUMA & STRESS DISORDERS
309.81 / F43.10 Post Traumatic Stress Disorder (PTSD)
- Severe Trauma - experienced trauma, witnessed trauma, or learned about violent trauma to loved one
- Intrusive memories, nightmares, flashbacks
- Avoidance - (avoid memories, thoughts, feelings, reminders)
- Negative thoughts & feelings: amnesia to the event, exaggerated negative beliefs, self (or other) blame, persistent fear / anger / horror / shame, low interest in activities, feeling detached, feeling numb
- Hyperarousal (insomnia, poor concentration, emotional lability, hypervigilance, exaggerated startle, reckless or self destructive behavior)
- Symptoms present for 1 month and work / social impairment

Preschool Subtype (under 6 years of age)

308.3 / F43.0 Acute Stress Disorder
- PTSD, but less than one month since trauma

Adjustment Disorders
- Stressor leading to excessive distress or work / social impairment
- Symptoms do not last greater than 6 months after resolution of stress
- Specify stress as acute or chronic (greater than 6 months)
309.0 / F43.21 Adjustment Disorders with depressed mood
309.24 / F43.22 Adjustment Disorders with anxiety
309.28 / F43.23 Adjustment Disorders with mixed anxiety and depressed mood
309.3 / F43.24 Adjustment Disorders with disturbance of conduct
309.4 / F43.25 Adjustment Disorders with mixed disturbance of emotions and conduct

313.89 / F94.1 Reactive Attachment Disorder
- Poor care-giving at early age (neglected, deprived, too numerous care-givers, or orphanage)
- Emotionally withdrawn behavior towards care-givers (doesn't seek or respond to comfort)
- Socially and emotionally unresponsive, inappropriately irritable / sad / or fearful

313.89 / F94.2 Disinhibited Social Engagement Disorder
- Poor care-giving at early age (neglected, deprived, too numerous care-givers, or orphanage)
- Child inappropriately approaches or is overly familiar with unknown adult

DISSOCIATIVE DISORDERS
300.14 / F44.81 Dissociative Identity Disorder (Multiple Personality)
- 2 or more distinct personalities recurrently take control
- Compartmentalization of information
- Marked distress or impairment

300.12 / F44.0 Dissociative Amnesia
- Trauma leading to inability to remember personal information
- Marked distress or impairment
- Specify if it includes **Dissociative Fugue (travel) 300.13 / F44.1**

300.6 / F48.1 Depersonalization / Derealization Disorder
- Recurrent subjective detachment (as if an "outside observer" or in a dream)
- Intact reality testing (not psychotic)
- Marked distress or impairment

EATING DISORDERS
307.1 Anorexia Nervosa
- Reducing food intake and refusal to maintain minimally healthy weight
- Strong fear of gaining weight or being "fat"
- Disturbance in body image (usually perceiving self as much heavier)
- Mild: BMI above 17, Moderate: BMI 16-16.99, Severe: BMI 15 - 15.99, Extreme: BMI <15

> **307.1 / F50.01 Restricting Type** - no binge eating or purging (purely uses fasting and exercising)

> **307.1 / F50.02 Binge / Purge type** - some binges or purging (vomiting, laxatives, etc)

307.51 / F50.2 Bulimia Nervosa
- Binge eating with minimal sense of control
- Purging or over exercising

307.51 / F50.8 Binge Eating Disorder
- Binge eating with minimal sense of control
- No purging or over exercising to try to compensate

FEEDING DISORDERS
307.59 / F50.8 Avoidant / Restrictive Food Intake Disorder
- Extreme food preferences leading to substantial psychosocial or nutritional problems

307.52 / F98.3 (children) / F50.8 (adults) Pica
- Eating non-food items for 1 month or more
- Inappropriate for age

307.53 / F98.21 Rumination Disorder
- Persistent regurgitation of food (may be re-chewed or spit out)

ELIMINATION DISORDERS
307.6 / F98.0 Enuresis - Loss of control of urine (day or night)

307.7 / F98.1 Encopresis - Loss of control of stool (with or without constipation)

NEUROCOGNITIVE DISORDERS
293.0 / F05 Delirium
- Quick onset disturbance in attention, orientation, and cognition (memory, language & perception)
- Evidence of a medical cause (substance intoxication or withdrawal, toxin, medication reaction, or other physical illness)
- May also be more specific in coding to specific cause

Major Neurocognitive Disorder
- Significant cognitive decline in one or more areas (learning and memory, language, executive functioning, complex attention, perceptual-motor, or social cognition)
- Interferes to the point of needing assistance
- Specify (and code) subtypes when possible: Alzheimer's, Vascular, Substance Induced, Traumatic Brain Injury, HIV Infection, Parkinson's Disease, Lewy Bodies, Prion Disease, and Huntington's Disease

Mild Neurocognitive Disorders
- Modest cognitive decline in one or more areas (learning and memory, language, executive functioning, complex attention, perceptual-motor, or social cognition)
- Does not interfere with functioning or independence
- Specify (and code) subtypes when possible: Alzheimer's, Vascular, Substance Induced, Traumatic Brain Injury, HIV Infection, Parkinson's Disease, Lewy Bodies, Prion Disease, and Huntington's Disease

DISRUPTIVE IMPULSE-CONTROL DISORDERS
313.81/ F91.3 Oppositional Defiant Disorder
- Angry, argumentative, vindictive or defiant behavior for 6 months
- Marked distress or impairment

312.89 / F91.9 Conduct Disorder
- Persistently violates other's rights or societal rules (hurting people or animals, property destruction, lying, theft, illegal activity)
- May code more specifically for Childhood or Adolescent onset

312.34 / F63.81 Intermittent Explosive Disorder
- Recurrent verbal or physical outbursts out of character for the person and disproportionate to the stress

312.32 / F63.3 Kleptomania
- Recurrent impulsive stealing of un-needed items
- Build up of tension prior to the act and relief following it

312.33 / F63.1 Pyromania
- Recurrent fire setting and attraction to fire
- Build up of tension prior to the act and relief following it

SOMATIC DISORDERS
300.82 / F45.1 Somatic Symptom Disorder
- Disproportionately excessive response (thoughts, feelings or behaviors) to a distressing physical symptom
- Usually persists at least 6 months

300.7 / F45.21 Illness Anxiety Disorder
- Excessive worry over having a serious illness, despite minimal medical evidence
- High anxiety around health overall
- Excessive health-related activities (symptom checking, tests, doctor visits, etc), or avoids medical care

316 / F54 Psychological Factors Affecting Medical Condition
- Psychological factors adversely affect the course of a medical illness

300.19 / F68.10 Factitious Disorder
- Intentional faking to achieve a sick role
- No clear economic or legal motivators

300.11 Conversion Disorder (Functional Neurological Symptom Disorder)
- Abnormal voluntary motor or sensory functioning
- Symptoms are incompatible with recognized neurologic or medical conditions
- Marked distress or impairment

Document Subtype:

F44.4: Weakness, paralysis, abnormal movement, swallowing, speech

F44.5: Seizures

F44.6: Anesthesia or sensory loss

F44.7: Mixed

SLEEP-WAKE DISORDERS

780.52 / G47.00 Insomnia Disorder
- Difficulty initiating or maintaining sleep, 3 nights a week for at least 3 months
- Marked distress or impairment

780.54 / G47.10 Hypersomnolence Disorder
- Excessive sleepiness despite sleeping at least 7 hours per night
- One of the following: non-restorative sleep lasting 9 hours or more, recurrent lapsing into sleep through the day, or difficulty awakening
- Occurs 3 times a week for at least 3 months
- Marked distress or impairment
- Not better explained by: sleep apnea, narcolepsy, parasomnias etc

Narcolepsy
- Irresistible sleep attacks, at least 3 times a week for 3 months
- At least one of the following:
  - Cataplexy: sudden loss of muscle tone after laughing
  - Hypocretin deficiency on spinal tap
  - Sleep study showing reduced REM sleep latency
- ICD 9 and 10 coded by specific subtypes

307.45 Circadian Rhythm Sleep-Wake Disorders
G47.21 - Delayed Sleep Phase
G47.22 - Advanced Sleep Phase
G47.23 - Irregular Sleep-wake Type
G47.24 - Non 24-hour Sleep-wake Type
G47.26 - Shift work type
G47.20 - Unspecified type

BREATHING RELATED SLEEP DISORDERS
327.23 / G47.33 Obstructive Sleep Apnea Hypopnea
– Diagnosed via sleep study

Central Sleep Apnea
– Diagnosed via sleep study
– ICD 9 and 10 coded by specific subtypes

Sleep-Related Hypoventilation
– Diagnosed via sleep study
– ICD 9 and 10 coded by specific subtypes

PARASOMNIAS
307.47 / F51.5 Nightmare Disorder
– Repeated terrifying awakenings with vivid recall and alertness
– Marked distress or impairment

327.42 / G47.52 Rapid Eye Movement Sleep Behavior Disorder
– Repeated sleep arousals with speaking or complex movements (walking, etc)
– Quickly awakens, fairly alert and not disoriented

333.94 / G25.81 Restless Legs Syndrome
– Urges to move legs, unpleasant restless sensation in legs, worse at night
– Occur at least 3 times a week for 3 months
– Marked distress or impairment

307.46 Non–REM Sleep Arousal Disorders
– No or little dream material recalled

   307.46 / F51.3 Sleepwalking type: blank stare, relatively unresponsive, hard to awaken, no dream recall

   307.46 / F51.4 Sleep Terror type: abrupt arousals, panic scream, intense fear and autonomic arousal

GENDER DYSPHORIA
302.6 / F64.9 Gender Dysphoria
- Conflict between one's assigned gender and their experience of their gender. A strong preference for characteristics of the opposite gender to which they were assigned.
- Clinically significant distress or impairment

SEXUAL DISORDERS
302.72 / F52.22 Female Sexual Interest / Arousal Disorder
- Absent or reduced sexual interest or arousal

302.72 / F52.21 Erectile Disorder

302.73 / F52.31 Female Orgasmic Disorder
- Delayed or absence of orgasm

302.74 / F52.32 Delayed Ejaculation

302.76 / F52.6 Genito-Pelvic Pain/Penetration Disorder

302.71 / F52.0 Male Hypoactive Sexual Desire Disorder

302.75 / F52.4 Premature (Early) Ejaculation

PARAPHILIC DISORDERS
302.4 / F65.2 Exhibitionistic Disorder
- Fantasies or behavior to expose genitals to unsuspecting others
- Marked distress or impairment

302.81 / F65.0 Fetishistic Disorder
- Intense sexual fantasies or behavior with non-living object or non-genital body part
- Marked distress or impairment

302.89 / F65.81 Frotteuristic Disorder
- Fantasies or behaviors of touching or rubbing again an unsuspecting adult
- Marked distress or impairment

302.2 / F65.4 Pedophilic Disorder
- Fantasies or behavior of sexual activity with a prepubescent child (usually 12 and under)
- The perpetrator is 16 years of age or older, and is 5 years older than victim
- Marked distress or impairment

302.83 / F65.51 Sexual Masochism Disorder
- Fantasies or behaviors of experiencing sexual humiliation or suffering
- Marked distress or impairment

302.84 / F65.52 Sexual Sadism Disorder
- Fantasies or behaviors of inflicting suffering on others
- Marked distress or impairment

302.3 / F65.1 Transvestic Disorder
- Fantasies or behaviors of cross-dressing
- Marked distress or impairment

302.82 / F65.3 Voyeuristic Disorder
- Arousal from observing unsuspecting person in sexual context or disrobed
- Marked distress or impairment

302.89 / F65.89 Other Specified Paraphilic Disorder
- Other paraphilias such as telephone scatologia (obscene calls), necrophilia (dead body), zoophilia (animals), coprophilia (feces), klismaphilia (enemas), urophilia, etc.
- Marked distress or impairment

PERSONALITY DISORDERS
Cluster A: "Odd" Group
301.0 / F60.0 Paranoid Personality Disorder
- Distrust since early adulthood
- 4 out of 7 symptoms: suspects deception, doubts loyalty of friends, reluctant to confide, reads hidden meanings, bears grudges, perceives personal attacks on character, unwarranted suspicions of partner

301.20 / F60.1 Schizoid Personality Disorder
- Detached social relationships
- 4 out of 7 symptoms: doesn't desire close relationships, solitary activities, no interest in a sex partner, few close friends, little pleasure in activities, indifferent to praise or criticism, emotional coldness or flat affect

301.22 / F21 Schizotypal Personality Disorder
- Eccentricities and few close relationships
- 5 out of 9 symptoms: odd behavior, magical thinking (ESP, superstitions), ideas of reference, illusions, odd thinking and speech, paranoia, inappropriate or constricted affect, few close friends, excessive social anxiety

Cluster B: "Dramatic" Group
301.83 / F60.3 Borderline Personality Disorder
- Unstable relationships, unstable self image, unstable affects and impulsivity
- 5 out of 9 symptoms: frantically avoids abandonment, idealizes then devalues relationships, identity disturbance, dangerous impulsivity, recurrent suicidal thoughts or self-mutilation, affective instability, chronic empty feeling, anger control problems, transient dissociation or paranoia

301.50 / F60.4 Histrionic Personality Disorder
- Excessive emotions and attention seeking
- 5 out of 8 symptoms: center of attention, sexually seductive, shallow and unstable emotions, dresses to draw attention, emotional speech without substance, theatrical, suggestible and easily influenced, feels relationships are more intimate then they really are

301.81 / F60.81 Narcissistic Personality Disorder
- Grandiosity, need for admiration and lack of empathy since early adulthood
- 5 out of 9 symptoms: grandiosity, fantasies of unlimited power and success, sees self as "special" and only associates with others of high status, needs admiration, sense of entitlement, interpersonally exploitative, lacks empathy, envious of others, arrogant

301.7 / F60.2 Antisocial Personality Disorder
- Evidence of conduct disorder before age 15
- Disregards other's rights since age 15
- 3 out of 7 symptoms: repeated unlawful acts, deceitfulness, impulsivity, repeated physical fights, disregard for safety, consistent irresponsibility, lack of remorse

Cluster C: "Withdrawn" Group
301.82 / F60.6 Avoidant Personality Disorder
- Inhibited, inadequate and hypersensitive
- 4 out of 7 symptoms: avoids occupations dealing with people, avoids people unless they'll be liked, restrained in close relationships, fears social rejection, social inhibition, feels socially inept, few new activities or risks

301.6 / F60.7 Dependent Personality Disorder
- Excessive need to be taken care of
- Submissive and clingy behavior
- Fears of separation
- 5 out of 8 symptoms: difficulty making decisions, doesn't take responsibility, avoids conflict, poor initiation of projects, craves nurturance, helpless when alone, urgently seeks out relationships when one ends, fears being left to take care of themselves

301.4 / F60.5 Obsessive-Compulsive Personality Disorder
- Orderly, perfectionistic and in control
- 4 out of 8 symptoms: overly preoccupied by details; interfering perfectionism, workaholic, overly strict values, pack rat, micromanages others, miserly, rigid and stubborn

ACKNOWLEDGEMENTS...

I am indebted to the many souls that have supported this book in coming into being.

My grounding and core has been my wife, Megan Reilly Buser. Her constant love and encouragement has been the wellspring of my creativity through the many years. I am grateful for my son, Brian Buser, and his dogged persistence in urging me to hire his friend and then 5th grade classmate, Luke Sloan, to illustrate this book. Luke's tireless work blended beautifully the purity of a child's eye with the budding wisdom of a young man. Luke's mother, Jeryl Sloan was a faithful courier of her son's precious artwork. I am grateful to Saila Buser for adding color both to my home as well as the cover illustration of our book. My co-author, Len Cruz, sculpted my words, adding his own thoughts to the book and together helped me fashion a finished manuscript. Finally, I remain indebted to Dr. Murray Stein, who has been my teacher, my mentor, and my friend. His influence is unfathomable. In all matters, I am indebted to Don and Joan Buser who have believed in me and nurtured me these many years.

- Steve Buser

SECTION I

OVERVIEW

CHAPTER 1

INTRODUCTION

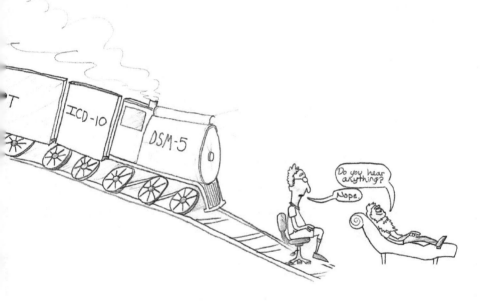

This book is for busy clinicians wishing to get a quick command of the various changes introduced in the new *Diagnostic and Statistical Manual Version 5* (DSM-5). The audience for this book includes therapists, psychiatrists, psychologists, counselors, physicians, residents in training, medical students, others in the mental health field, and interested laypersons.

We make liberal use of cartoons and hyperbole in order to capture broad ideas. We ask the reader's indulgence in recognizing that these conventions do not capture the nuance and subtle features that so often accompany people into the consulting room. The authors hope that by presenting engaging cartoons that attempt to reduce complex ideas into easily remembered images, the process of transition from earlier versions of the DSM to the present one will be made easier.

Beginning as early as 2015, the ICD-10 (International Statistical Classification of Diseases and Related Health Problems) codes are expected to be adopted by all healthcare providers in the United States. Throughout this book ICD-10 is used. Combined with Appendix 1, the authors hope to familiarize clinicians with the changes that are awaited in 2015. Certain devices are used to assist the reader in remembering principles and ideas.

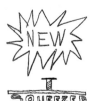 This signifies a newly created diagnosis or category.

 This signifies that things have been condensed/compressed.

 This signifies an expansion of a category.

 This signifies that something has been moved (often unchanged).

~~~~~~~~~~~~~~~~

I'm interested in themes that endure from generation to generation.

                                                DAVID GUTERSON

GENERATIONS OF DSM

The DSM-5 arrived 20 years after its predecessor, DSM-IV. That is a generation in the human family. The DSM-IV had embedded itself in the very fabric of how mental illness is conceptualized and it had influenced what it means to enjoy mental health.

The DSM-5 remains a symptom-driven system of classification. At the National Institute of Mental Health, some people have expressed an intention to move away from the DSM's symptom-based approach in favor of a greater focus on biology, genetics, and neuroscience. [1] According to Thomas Insel,

> *We are committed to new and better treatments, but we feel this will only happen by developing a more precise diagnostic system.*[2]

An alternate schema would likely emphasize putative (presumed) causation over presenting symptoms.

Chapter 2 provides a historical overview of DSM-5. This chapter also provides a conceptual framework whereby mental illness is understood to exist along a continuum of severity and presenting symptoms. We propose 8 key groupings of mental illness that easily lend themselves to this *Spectrum* approach. Within each of these groupings, a spectrum of severity and functioning is presented. Each *Spectrum* is depicted with a mnemonic device, a cartoon, which also introduces the Jungian idea of *enantiodromia*. This is a principle introduced by C. G. Jung that describes a phenomenon whereby any force that manifests in excess inevitably produces its opposite, albeit in the unconscious.[3]

Chapter 3 provides a survey of what is new in DSM-5. This chapter emphasizes the idea that mental disorders exist along a *Spectrum*. For example, Bipolar Disorder is no longer approached in quite so black and white a fashion. With earlier versions of the DSM patients either met criteria or they failed to meet criteria for the diagnosis. This approach may have led some clinicians to embellish findings in order to qualify a patient for a diagnosis or ignore certain criteria in order to assign a patient more benign appearing diagnosis.

Chapter 4 introduces the central idea of this book - *8 Primary Spectrums of Mental Illness*. These *8 Spectrums of Mental Illness* are covered in more detail in Chapters 5 through 12. A chapter is devoted to each of the *8 Primary Spectrum of Mental Illness*. Each *Spectrum* provides a simplified, useful framework for clinicians to approach the DSM-5's new *spectrum* approach to diagnosis. For example, when considering *Bipolarity* a person situated at the extreme end of the spectrum will demonstrate a full complement of symptoms associated with Bipolar Affective Disorder in the manic phase (see Chapter 6). At the other extreme of *Bipolarity*, a depressed person would be noted to be thoroughly lacking in creativity, risk-taking, and verve.

A cartoon caricature depicting each of the *8 Spectrums of Mental Illnesses* is intended to anchor in the reader's memory one prominent feature of each diagnostic category. In the middle of each scale there appears a large territory in which most people would hope to dwell. This is the domain typically considered healthy, normal functioning.

Chapter 13 addresses most of the remaining diagnoses that appear in DSM-5. We assign them to a secondary category, neither because they are of lesser importance nor because they cause less disruption to the sufferer. With the possible exception of Trauma, the disorders covered in Chapter 13 may simply occur less frequently or clinicians may be less likely to encounter these disorders in daily practice. Trauma is covered in Chapter 13 because it did not lend itself as readily to the spectrum approach used. The convention of using a scale of severity has not been extended to the conditions covered in Chapter 13. The Chapter-13 disorders include Trauma- and Stressor-Related Disorders, Dissociative Disorders, Somatic Symptom and Related Disorders, Feeding and Eating Disorders, Elimination Disorders, Sleep–Wake Disorders, Sexual Dysfunctions, Gender Dysphoria, Neurocognitive Disorders, and Paraphilic Disorders.

Chapter 14, *The Harmony of the Lotus Flower,* emerges from the concept of *8 Spectrums of Mental Illness.* The *Lotus* comprises the *8 Primary Spectrums of Mental Illness* folded in on one another to create the image of a flower. This chapter is unabashedly Jungian in its perspective. The centermost realm where these spectrums intersect is imagined as the realm where balance, *conjunctio oppositurum* (conjunction of opposites), and harmony is most often and most easily secured. Chaos and symptoms arise on the periphery of the lotus flower whereas the center holds things together. When a person manifests the features located in the center of the *Lotus* the archetypal *SELF may* find its optimum expression.

Those familiar with quantum mechanics may recall the idea of complementarity wherein a subatomic particle's position and velocity cannot both be precisely determined. Precise measurement of a particle's speed results in the blurring of its possible positions.

This can also be represented as a blurry collection of probability waves. This metaphor fits nicely with the elusive exercise of establishing a diagnosis. It reminds all clinicians that we can never locate a person with complete precision. Chapter 15 offers another Jungian perspective on DSM-5. We indulge in a bit of *active imagination* of our own in which Jung is confronted with DSM-5. It should be kept in mind that Jung began his career as a solid researcher and his discoveries using the word association test is what helped inform him of the unique features of the unconscious.

The Appendix introduces ICD-10 codes that apply to psychiatry, psychology, and other mental health disciplines. The Centers for Medicare & Medicaid Services (CMS) extended the deadline for implementation of ICD-10 until October 1, 2015. The ICD-10-CM uses 3 to 7 digits instead of the 3 to 5 digits used with ICD-9 and the coding is more specific than in ICD-9. Beginning October 1, 2015, all healthcare services provided in the United States must use ICD-10 codes unless another delay is introduced.

CHAPTER 2

THE HISTORY OF THE DSM

Many different systems of classifying mental illness have been developed throughout history. To varying degrees these systems tended to emphasize: presenting symptoms, presumed causes, and distinguishing features between disorders. Because different systems of diagnosis and nomenclature emphasized different things, translation between different systems proved difficult. *DSM-5 Insanely Simplified: Unlocking the Spectrums within DSM-5 & ICD-10* attempts to make the translation between DSM-IV and DSM-5 easier while introducing *ICD-10*. What follows is a brief history of different systems of classification.

ANTIQUITY

Hippocrates recognized distinct categories of mental illness that included melancholia, mania, and paranoia. An ancient theory of causation was that imbalances of humors produced mental disturbances.

PERSIA AND THE MUSLIM EMPIRE

Arabic and Persian scholars translated the works of the Greeks and Romans. These scholars expanded the diagnostic categories to include delusional disorders, anger and aggression, and other disorders. The QUR'ĀN advises against entrusting to the *insane* material belongings given by Allah, but it goes on to instruct that such persons be fed and clothed with the property that belongs to them.[4] The first psychiatric hospital was established in Baghdad in 705 AD. Jinn, spiritual creatures who can possess a person, were often thought to be the cause of mental illness.

EARLY CHRISTENDOM

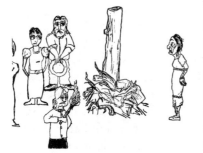

While early European Christendom distinguished between *idiocy* and *lunacy*, causation was commonly ascribed to evil forces. By the close of the 17th century, mental illness was being recognized as an organic disorder; yet madhouses continued to treat their inmates like wild beasts in need of taming. Bedlam, the most notorious of the madhouses, charged spectators to watch the inmates.

19TH CENTURY AND BEYOND

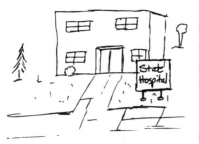

Dorthea Dix campaigned for better treatment of the mentally ill. She petitioned the government of the United States to build large institutions to house people. Eventually, 32 State psychiatric hospitals were established around the country. The 19th century also witnessed the introduction of familiar terms like obsession neurosis, agoraphobia, somatization disorder, kleptomania, pyromania, and psychopathic inferiority.

STATISTICAL MANUAL FOR THE USE OF INSTITUTIONS FOR THE INSANE (1844-1917)

Beginning in 1844, the forerunner of the American Psychiatric Association compiled statistical information about patients living in mental institutions around the nation. In 1917, a committee on statistics produced a report that included 22 separate diagnoses.

DSM-I RELEASED IN 1952 (ORIGINAL PRICE $3.90)

The first DSM was produced in 1952 and was based largely on the nomenclature used by psychiatrists in World War II. It sought to coincide with ICD-6. It was 130 pages in length and included 106 mental disorders. It introduced the idea of "reaction," in part, due to the influence of Adolph Meyer, a University of Zürich trained American psychiatrist who advanced the notion of a biopsychosocial model of understanding psychopathology. The DSM-I distinguished personality disturbance from neurosis.

DSM-II RELEASED IN 1968

The DSM-II expanded the number of diagnoses to 182. The influence of psychodynamic principles was evident in the broad distinction made between neurosis and psychosis. The DSM-II tried to strive toward an "atheoretical" approach. The DSM-II was designed to conform to ICD-8. Harking back to antiquity where homosexuality had been referred to as *Scythians Disease,* homosexuality was considered a Mental Disorder. This changed in 1974.

DSM-III RELEASED IN 1980 (ORIGINAL PRICE $25.00)

The DSM-III introduced the multiaxial system of diagnoses and it conformed to ICD-9.

The Multiaxial System:
Axis I: Clinical Disorders of Mental Illness
Axis II: Personality Disorders and Mental Retardation
Axis III: General Medical Conditions
Axis IV: Psychosocial and Environmental Problems (homelessness, legal issues, etc.)
Axis V: Global Assessment of Functioning: A single number from 0 to 100

There was a clear shift away from a psychodynamic approach. In the place of psychodynamic approaches a biopsychosocial model rose in prominence. The DSM-III grew to 494 pages and recognized 265 diagnoses. A problem that arose with the DSM-III was the all-or-nothing approach to diagnosis. A specific number of symptoms had to be established in order to meet criteria for a diagnosis.

DSM-III-R RELEASED IN 1987

This revision made modest changes in the organization of DSM-III and made changes in criteria. The number of diagnoses rose to 292 and the book expanded to 567 pages.

DSM-IV RELEASED IN 1994 (ORIGINAL PRICE $65.00)

The DSM-IV changed very little; nevertheless, it expanded to 886 pages and added 5 more disorders to reach a total of 297 disorders. It conformed to ICD-9. Considerable controversy was provoked by the publication of DSM-III and this led to an exhaustive amount of literature review, extensive review of data compiled using DSM-III, and 13 work groups were called upon to manage specific sections.

DSM-IV-TR RELEASED IN 2000 (ORIGINAL PRICE $84.00)

TR "Text Revision" corrected minor errors and improved the supportive educational material. It also made some additional refinements to assure conformity with the ICD-9 system.

DSM-5 $199.00 ($149.00 PAPERBACK)

The work to revise DSM-IV began in 1999. Once again, 13 working groups were established. An enormous amount of money, $3 million, was spent on what proved to be useless field-testing. The thrust of DSM-5 was designed to usher in a system of classification wherein mental disorders exist along a spectrum. **DSM-5 strives** to be **evidence-based**. There was an attempt to eliminate the category of Not Otherwise Specified (NOS). DSM-5 appeared just prior to the original dates when ICD-10 was supposed to be implemented. The transition from ICD-9 to ICD-10 was delayed once more and the new date for implementation became October 1, 2015; therefore, both codes appeared in DSM-5. The DSM-5 is 992 pages in length.

CHAPTER 3

WHAT IS NEW IN DSM-5?

Many things in DSM-5 will seem familiar to clinicians accustomed to DSM-IV despite the drastic revisions. The first thing clinicians will notice is the **removal of the Multi-axial System** of diagnosis (Axis I, II, III, IV, V). In its place, there is an attempt to shift toward conceptualizing mental illness along a spectrum of severity while also encouraging more of a developmental approach.

Woven into the very fabric of DSM-5 is a concept that mental illness exists along a **spectrum** of functioning and severity, from very minimal or "normal" levels to more extreme "pathologic" symptoms.

DSM-5 makes less clear distinction between "normal" and "mentally ill". Chapter 4 explores, in more detail, this paradigm shift in DSM-5 of "illness as a spectrum" phenomenon that overarches the latest DSM.

DSM-5 utilizes 2 new terms, **Subtypes** and **Specifiers,** to further refine diagnostic impressions. Keep in mind that Subtypes are mutually exclusive whereas Specifiers are not mutually exclusive and are noted as "*Specify*" or "*Specify* if".

When using DSM-5 in an **inpatient setting** the **Principal diagnosis** is understood to be the one "chiefly responsible for occasioning the admission of the individual."[5] **Provisional Diagnosis** is intended for circumstances where either the duration or the full criteria have not yet been met but are expected to be met.

DSM-5 introduces several other changes. There are a number of other changes in the new DSM-5:

DEPRESSION (MOOD DISORDERS)

> *"In itself pain will sanctify no man: it may even tend to wrap him up within himself, and make him morose, peevish, selfish; but when God blesses it, then it will have a most salutary effect—a supplying, softening influence."*
>
> CHARLES SPURGEON, 1881 SERMON.[6]

Depression has been described as the gout of the soul. Like gout, it recurs, it causes intense discomfort, and in between flare-ups there often exists little evidence that it ever visited. DSM-III introduced the diagnosis of Dysthymic Disorder or Dysthymia. This term *Dysthymia*, coined by Dr. Robert Spitzer who chaired the task force that developed DSM-III, replaced the psychoanalytically-oriented term, "neurotic depression". Years later, Dr. Spitzer expressed reservations about how DSM-III had medicalized the normal human experience.

The distinguishing feature of **Dysthymic Disorder** was a depressive disorder lasting **at least 2 years** that failed to meet the full criteria of a Major Depression. **Persistent Depressive Disorder** replaces Dysthymic Disorder and subsumes the category of Recurrent Major Depression. The result is that the persistent quality of the depression replaces severity as a defining feature.

The **Mixed Features Specifiers** allow clinicians to document the presence of significant **bipolarity**. Similarly, the **Anxiety Specifiers** allow significant anxiety components to be documented. In earlier versions of the DSM the presence of bereavement excluded the diagnosis of depression; this is no longer the case. Patients who are actively grieving may be diagnosed with depression. Finally, DSM-5 introduces a **new disorder** to this category, **Premenstrual Dysphoric Disorder**.

BIPOLAR DISORDER (MOOD DISORDERS)

Greater emphasis is placed upon **increased energy** and **increased activity level** with less emphasis being given to the specific valence of the person's mood (i.e., expansive, euphoric, irritable). Bipolar diagnosis can include **Mixed Features Specifiers** that allow clinicians to document significant **Depressive features** and **Anxiety Specifiers**.

ANXIETY DISORDERS

DSM-5 **removes OCD** (Obsessive Compulsive Disorder) and **PTSD** (Post Traumatic Stress Disorder) from the section of Anxiety Disorders. They are placed among 2 newly created categories of **OCD and Related Disorders** and **Trauma Stress Disorders** respectively.

Two diagnoses have been moved to the Anxiety Disorders; **Separation Anxiety Disorder** and **Selective Mutism** have been moved from the category of "Disorders of Childhood".

DSM-5 distinguishes **Panic Disorder** and **Agoraphobia** as 2 **distinct** disorders. Recognizing that **Panic Attacks** appear in the presence of various other disorders, clinicians may use **Panic Attack Specifier**. This also makes clear that a Panic Attack is **not** a mental disorder, per se.

PSYCHOSIS (SCHIZOPHRENIA AND OTHER PSYCHOTIC DISORDERS)

The **5 subtypes** of **Schizophrenia** (catatonic, disorganized, paranoid, residual, and undifferentiated) no longer characterize this disorder. Instead, **Catatonia** is now a **Specifier** and can be employed with Schizophrenia, Bipolar Disorder, and Depression. At least **1 positive symptom** (hallucinations, delusions, or disorganized speech) is now **required** to meet the criteria for Schizophrenia. **Schizoaffective Disorder requires** that either depression or bipolar features be present for a majority of the disorder's duration.

OBSESSIVE COMPULSIVE AND RELATED DISORDERS

Stretched DSM-5 adds a new group of disorders known as the OCD and Related Disorders. This includes not only what has traditionally been **OCD** itself, but certain related illnesses including: **Body Dysmorphic Disorder** and **Trichotillomania**. Newly created diagnoses in this section are **Excoriation Disorder** (skin picking) and **Hoarding Disorder**. *If cable television recognizes hoarding as a disorder then certainly DSM-5's inclusion of the disorder is overdue, right?*

SUBSTANCE ABUSE DISORDERS

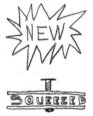 **No distinction** is made between Substance **Abuse** and Substance **Dependence**. This is in keeping with the "Spectrum" approach. The main diagnostic heading is Substance Abuse Disorder. The various substances of abuse are now subsumed under this heading: **Criteria.**

Criteria 1–4	Craving
Criteria 5–7	Impaired Social Functioning
Criteria 8–9	Failure to Consider Risks of Use
Criterion 10	Tolerance
Criterion 11	Withdrawal

DSM-5 recognizes that **craving** is a hallmark feature of Substance Abuse Disorders and the first group of Criteria 1–4 reflect this. Impaired social functioning is established with Criteria 5–7. The failure to consider the risks of use is reflected in Criteria 8–9. Criterion 10 addresses tolerance—the phenomenon whereby an increasing dose of a substance is required to produce a desired effect. Criterion 11 addresses withdrawal—the physiologic phenomenon whereby symptoms arise upon abrupt cessation of a substance that has been used for a prolonged time. Note that neither tolerance nor withdrawal is required to establish the diagnosis. The criterion of "recurrent substance-related legal problems" has been removed.

 Gambling Disorder is recognized in DSM-5 as sharing sufficient features in common with Substance Abuse Disorders as to warrant inclusion in this category.

The substances include: **Alcohol, Caffeine, Cannabis, Hallucinogen, Opioids, Sedative-Hypnotics/Anxiolytics, Stimulants, Tobacco, and Other.**

The **Severity** may be described as mild, moderate, or severe depending upon the number of criteria that are met. Clinicians can specify whether **intoxication** or **withdrawal** is involved (think of this as Specifiers).

 Tobacco Use Disorder has also been **added.**

NEURODEVELOPMENTAL DISORDERS

The Neurodevelopmental Disorders first appear in childhood and are capable of producing lasting impairment of academic, social, occupational, and intrapersonal functioning. The disorders include: **Autism Spectrum Disorder** (ASD), **Attention Deficit Hyperactivity Disorder** (ADHD), **Communication Disorder, Specific Learning Disorder, and Motor Disorders.**

 DSM-5 conflates Autism, Asperger's Disorder, Childhood Disintegrative Disorder, and Pervasive Developmental Disorder NOS into one diagnosis called **Autism Spectrum Disorder** (ASD). Asperger's Disorder, previously viewed as less stigmatizing, is now officially an ASD.

ASD is characterized by 1) deficits in social communication and social interaction and 2) restricted repetitive behaviors. Where only social communication and interaction is impaired, the diagnosis should be Social Communication Disorder.

ADHD is virtually unchanged.

Specific Learning Disorder replaces Reading Disorder, Mathematics Disorder, and Disorder of Written Expression and clinicians should specify if any of the above features are present. The diagnosis of **Mental Retardation** has been **replaced** by **Intellectual Developmental Disorder**. This disorder is now assessed more by adaptive functioning and less by absolute IQ score.

PERSONALITY DISORDERS

DSM-5 abolishes Axis II. DSM-5 has not removed the Personality Disorders; the diagnosis is simply listed like any other disorder. The criteria for personality disorders are virtually unchanged in DSM-5. All 10 personality disorders from DSM-IV are carried over into DSM-5.

TRAUMA-RELATED DISORDERS

 DSM-5 establishes a new section for Trauma and Stressor Related Disorders. These include: **PTSD, Acute Stress Disorder, Adjustment Disorders,** and **Reactive Attachment Disorder.** PTSD introduces a new cluster of symptoms pertaining to negative changes in an individual's mood and cognition. "Negative alterations in cognitions and mood associated with the traumatic event."[7] This addresses the features of lacunae or holes in memory about traumatic events along with exaggeration, diminishing, distortion, and impaired emotional life that appear so commonly with trauma. Allowances are made for **indirect exposure** to a traumatic event.

If **Dissociative Symptoms** are present, the clinician should specify with Dissociative Symptoms. Special mention is made **for Posttraumatic Stress Disorder for Children 6 Years and Younger. Adjustment disorder,** by definition results from stress and therefore was moved to the category of Trauma- and Stressor-Related Disorders.

NEUROCOGNITIVE DISORDERS

DSM-5 introduces a substantial shift in the diagnostic schema regarding Dementia. The term **Dementia** has been **replaced** with **Neurocognitive Disorder** (NCD). Here too, a **spectrum** of functioning is recognized by distinguishing **Mild** NCDs from **Major** NCDs. The Neurocognitive Disorders include a long list of subtypes that are distinguished from one another by the specific cause of the disorder. **Subtypes** include: Alzheimer's, Vascular, Substance Induced, Traumatic Brain Injury, HIV Infection, Parkinson's Disease, Lewy Bodies, Prion Disease, and Huntington's Disease.

DISSOCIATIVE DISORDERS (DISSOCIATIVE DISORDERS)

Dissociative Disorders are listed as a separate diagnostic category that includes: **Dissociative Identity Disorder, Dissociative Amnesia, Depersonalization/Derealization Disorder** (this subsumed Depersonalization Disorder). **Dissociative Fugue** is no longer a distinct diagnosis but is a **Specifier.**

SOMATIC SYMPTOM DISORDER (SOMATOFORM DISORDERS)

Somatic Symptom Disorder is a new diagnostic construct in DSM-5. Somatization Disorder, Hypochondriasis, Pain Disorder, and Undifferentiated Somatoform Disorder have all been removed and replaced by the new Somatic Symptom Disorder diagnosis. This disorder essentially considers the degree to which a patient with any physical symptoms is experiencing excessively distressing feelings, thoughts, or behaviors beyond what the physical symptoms would typically cause. This new diagnosis eliminates the requirement of "unexplained medical symptoms," which so often angered patients who felt they were being accused of "just making it up!"

FEEDING AND EATING DISORDERS

 This is a new nomenclature in DSM-5. The diagnoses of Pica and Rumination Disorder are no longer restricted to childhood and can now be made at any age. A **new** disorder, **Avoidant/ Restrictive Food Intake Disorder**, is primarily confined to **children** who have extreme food preferences leading to substantial psychological or nutritional problems. In women, **Anorexia Nervosa** no longer requires amenorrhea. The frequency of purging behavior required to diagnose **Bulimia Nervosa** has been reduced from twice per week to once per week. When overeating with a loss of control and significant distress occurs at least weekly for 3 months, a new disorder, **Binge-Eating Disorder** is introduced.

SLEEP-WAKE DISORDER (SLEEP DISORDERS)

Sleep disorders often arise in conjunction with other medical or neurological conditions. The DSM-5 recommends that these disorders be understood as either being "lumped together" (as with insomnia) or "split apart" (as with narcolepsy) where validators exist. Primary Insomnia has been renamed as Insomnia Disorder. Under the category of Breathing-Related Sleep Disorders DSM-5 lists Obstructive Sleep Apnea, Central Sleep Apnea, and a new diagnosis of Sleep-Related Hypoventilation.

 Other **new** sleep disorders include **Rapid Eye Movement Sleep Behavior Disorder** and **Restless Leg Syndrome.**

GENDER DYSPHORIA (GENDER IDENTITY DISORDERS)

 Substantial changes in the attitudes toward persons who are Lesbian, Gay, Bisexual, Transgendered, or Queer (LGBTQ) over the past 20 years since the release of DSM-IV have been observed. In fact, largely due to the efforts of Dr. Robert Spitzer, homosexuality was removed from DSM-III and was no longer considered to be a mental illness. Gender Dysphoria is no longer deemed an "identity disorder". Gender incongruence results in dysphoria and difficulties in adapting.

Gender Dysphoria is no longer categorized alongside sexual dysfunctions and paraphilias. It is now segregated as its own category.

SEXUAL DYSFUNCTIONS

DSM-5 reorganizes the section of Sexual Dysfunctions. **Genito-Pelvic Pain/Penetration Disorder** replaces **Vaginismus** and **Dyspareunia**. Furthermore, the diagnosis of **Sexual Aversion Disorder** has been removed due to a lack of research evidence.

8 PRIMARY PSYCHIATRIC SPECTRUMS OF MENTAL ILLNESS

A major shift occurs with the introduction of DSM-5 that has broad implication for the way psychiatric illness is conceptualized. DSM-5 introduces the notion that illness exists along a spectrum or continuum rather than as an either/or phenomenon.

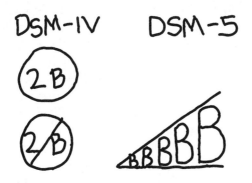

The DSM-5 planning groups established this idea from the outset, and throughout the manual the emphasis on illness as a spectrum is apparent. Also, the boundaries between certain disorders are less sharply defined in DSM-5. For example, Depression can have Bipolar or Anxiety "Specifiers" thereby acknowledging the overlap of the illness. Likewise, *Anxiety* disorder can be assigned *Bipolar* or *Depression* Specifiers. ASD incorporates the idea into its very name thereby drawing attention away from the idea that separate, discrete disorders exist. Likewise, under the heading of Substance Use Disorders, DSM-5 focuses upon using criteria to establish the level of severity rather than to determine the presence or absence of a disorder. Chapter 3 highlighted various examples of where the concept of illness along a spectrum makes an appearance in DSM-5. This chapter takes this concept one step further by simplifying and encapsulating DSM-5 into *The 8 Primary Spectrums of Psychiatry.*

CONSTRUCTING PRIMARY SPECTRUMS OF MENTAL ILLNESS

Everything should be made as simple as possible, but not simpler.

ALBERT EINSTEIN

We developed *The 8 Primary Spectrums of Mental Illness* as a tool to improve understanding. The *Spectrums* are not strictly based upon a collection or grouping of symptoms in the style of DSM-IV. We recognize that a great deal of work was done to develop DSM-5. Any attempt to simplify DSM-5 risks undermining some of the considerable work done to develop DSM-5. However, the DSM-5 speaks for itself; this guide is intended to enhance the usefulness of the DSM-5's very rich content. There is a real danger of oversimplifying the complexities of mental illness into tidy constructs. Diagnosis is not an easy art and should be approached with humility and respect for the complexities of the human condition. The following advice is offered:

The map is not the territory.

ALFRED KORZYBSKI

The clinician or lay person reading this book is advised to view these concepts as a broad approach. Beware to not impose them on patients. Beware that in making diagnoses you do not become too much like *Procrustes,* a rogue blacksmith who was intent on making travelers fit his iron bed by either stretching them or cutting off their legs. People are NOT their diagnoses.

Despite these pitfalls the core constructs offered here may give clinicians an easy, *big picture* approach to diagnosis as well as a means of monitoring the therapeutic process.

THE 8 PRIMARY SPECTRUMS OF MENTAL ILLNESS

The Depression Spectrum: Shallowness versus Despair
The Mania Spectrum: Boring versus Bipolar
The Anxiety Spectrum: Carelessness versus Anxiousness
The Psychosis Spectrum: Visionless versus Psychotic
The Focusing Spectrum: Attention Deficit Disorder versus Obsessive Compulsive Disorders
The Substance Abuse Spectrum: Ascetic versus Addicted
The Autism Spectrum: Codependent versus Autistic
The Personality Spectrum: Neurotic versus Obnoxious

Within each of these categories there exists a spectrum. At the extremes of the spectrums problems emerge. The middle ranges of these spectrums are preferable. The extreme ranges, where symptoms of mental illness appear, tend to interfere with life. The authors' views are strongly influenced by the work of Dr. C. G. Jung and his idea of *coniunctio oppositorum*, meaning the psychological conjunction of opposites.

DSM-5 diagnosis concerns itself with the extreme ends of these spectrums. The middle of each spectrum is a zone of "healthy functioning". The power of this spectrum approach is that clinicians no longer must fit patients into either a category of "healthy" or "disordered". Instead, gradations along a spectrum allow for more varied, nuanced understanding of the individual. While the boundaries between normal and ill become less clear, clinicians are granted more latitude. When symptoms begin interfering with normal functioning a line is crossed that leads to diagnosis of an illnesses and treatment.

The question facing clinicians now becomes not "does a person have bipolar disorder or not," but rather "how much bipolarity does a person have?." Everyone has some degree of bipolarity, for example, when overtaken by a surge of creativity, artistry, spontaneity, energy, sociability, talkativeness, and excitement. It is only when these features are "out of control" or produce negative consequences that a person enters the realm of what DSM-5 considers a "disorder."

Consider some ideas that derive from the concept of spectrums of illness.[8] How much Depressive-ness or Introspective-ness does a person have? How much Anxious-ness, OCD-ness, ADD-ness, Psychotic-ness, Addicted-ness, etc.

At first glance, it may seem that the ideal situation exists when a person shows as few characteristics as possible. However, the person displaying too few characteristics may have problems just like the person displaying excess. The *8 Primary Spectrums of Mental Illness* use a consistent convention whereby the left end of the spectrum represents the state of showing no features *(this is a problem)* and the right end of the spectrum represents the state of excessive features or symptoms *(this is also a problem)*.

This concept may become empowering to patients suffering symptoms of mental illness. One implication of a spectrum approach is that features manifesting in extreme forms constitute symptoms whereas in their attenuated form, the same features may be adaptive and desirable. "Normal" and "Abnormal" can be understood as states, not traits. Returning to normal may appear more attainable.

Everyone falls somewhere along the 8 spectrums. This conceptual model tends to destigmatize mental illness and strip it of shame. Just as the patient is located along a spectrum so are other people in their life. Everyone exists on a spectrum of severity or paucity of features. It may help to be reminded that we are all in this boat together.

Before proceeding to the more detailed presentation of the *8 Spectrums of Mental Illness* spend a few minutes reflecting on the following 8 illustrations. This will provide a visual introduction to the overarching concepts.

Shallowness vs. Despair
"How much SORROW do you hold?"

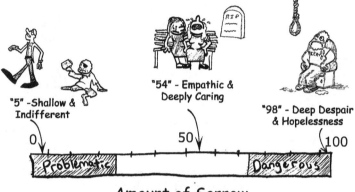

Amount of Sorrow

Boring vs. Bipolar
"How much CREATIVITY do you have?"

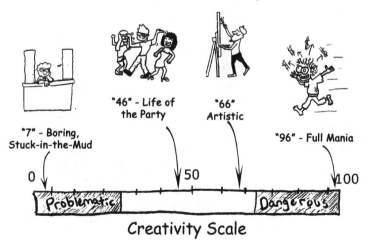

Creativity Scale

Carelessness vs. Anxiousness
"How much VIGILANCE do you have?"

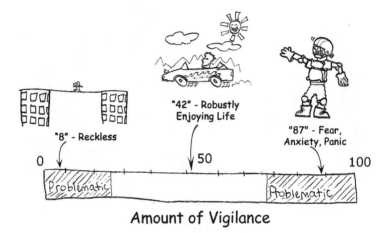

"8" - Reckless

"42" - Robustly
Enjoying Life

"87" - Fear,
Anxiety, Panic

0

50

100

Problematic

Problematic

Amount of Vigilance

Visionless vs. Psychotic:
"How strong are your DREAMS and VISIONS?"

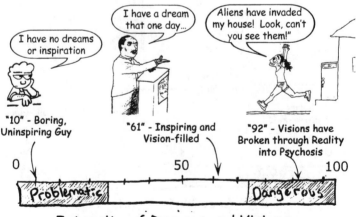

I have no dreams
or inspiration

I have a dream
that one day...

Aliens have invaded
my house! Look, can't
you see them!"

"10" - Boring,
Uninspiring Guy

"61" - Inspiring and
Vision-filled

"92" - Visions have
Broken through Reality
into Psychosis

0

50

100

Problematic

Dangerous

Intensity of Dreams and Visions

Attention Deficit Disorder (ADHD)
vs. Obsessive Compulsive Disorder (OCD)
"How much FOCUS do you have?"

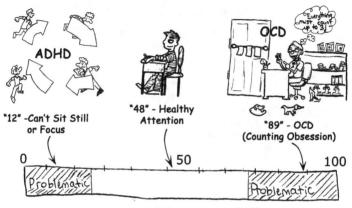

Amount of Focusing Ability

Ascetic Monk vs. Multiple Addictions:
"How Much PLEASURE Do You Seek?"

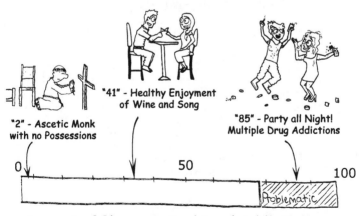

Amount of Pleasure Seeking / Addictiveness

Autism vs. Codependency:
How CONNECTED to Others are you?

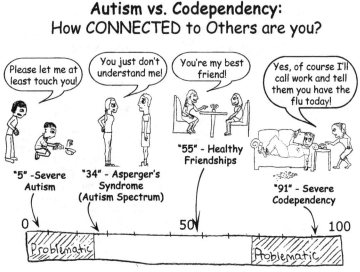

Degree of Connectedness to Others

Neurotic vs. Obnoxious:
"How much BLAME do you cast?"

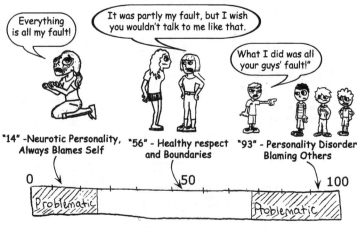

Amount of Blame Cast to Others

SECTION II

THE 8 PRIMARY SPECTRUMS OF PSYCHIATRY

CHAPTER 5

THE DEPRESSION SPECTRUM: SHALLOWNESS VERSUS DESPAIR (DEPRESSIVE DISORDERS)

DEPRESSION-WHAT'S NEW IN DSM-5

The concept of chronicity in *Depressive Disorders* changes in DSM-5. *Dysthymia,* a smoldering mild to moderate depression that presumably never meets the criteria for *Major Depression* and lasts at least 2 years has been eliminated. In its place is the diagnosis of **Persistent Depressive Disorder** that now **subsumes** chronic *Major Depression* as well as Dysthymic Disorder.

The distinguishing feature in DSM-5 is the chronic, *Persistent* nature of the mood disturbance. The degree of severity is de-emphasized while the degree of persistence is given priority. This reflects the common clinical presentation of recurring mood disorders. Severity often fluctuates dramatically while the persistence of melancholy remains a hallmark. Clinicians are permitted to include all the variations and tones of depressed mood together provided they demonstrate the feature of *persistence.*

In addition, clinicians can utilize **Mixed features specifiers** to **document** depression with significant **bipolarity**. Similarly, **Anxiety specifiers** allow clinicians to **document** depression with significant **anxiety** components. Furthermore, bereavement is no longer an exclusionary criterion for the diagnosis of depression. Actively grieving patients can also be diagnosed with depression.

Furthermore, 2 new diagnoses were added to the depression category in DSM-5, namely, *Premenstrual Dysphoric Disorder* and *Disruptive Mood Dysregulation Disorder.* Controversy has surrounded this disorder for years. In 1914, Lita Stetter Hollingsworth sought to establish that women were not impaired as a result of their menstrual cycles.[9] The controversy around this disorder continues.[10]

Premenstrual Dysphoric Disorder involves depressive symptoms in women occurring in the final week before onset of menses with improvement beginning shortly after menses begins. The remainder of the menstrual cycle is either free of symptoms or symptoms are minimal.

Disruptive Mood Dysregulation Disorder (Must be evidenced between Age 6–10) is characterized by severe and persistent irritability. This new diagnostic category involves frequent outbursts combined with a persistent angry/irritable backdrop. Onset must be prior to age 10 years.

DEPRESSION AS A SPECTRUM OF ILLNESS

As DSM-5 strives to introduce the concept of illness along a spectrum, black and white distinctions are abandoned in favor of a gradation of functioning and severity of presentation. Let's remember that a certain degree of sadness and depression is part of everyday life; along the spectrum there is a domain that shall be construed as normal.

The shallow, indifferent individual will tend to engage in limited or no introspection. Such a person might have difficulty learning from their mistakes. In contrast, the deeply despairing person tends to engage in an endless brooding sort of introspection. Such an individual may mull things over to such an exaggerated degree as to become paralyzed and feel crushed by their ceaseless ruminations and regurgitations of the past. In the middle, an individual

Shallowness vs. Despair
"How much SORROW do you hold?"

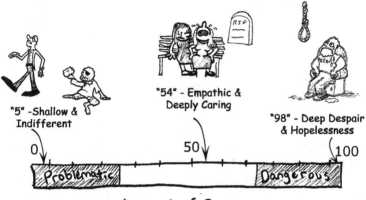

"54" - Empathic &
Deeply Caring

"5" -Shallow &
Indifferent

"98" - Deep Despair
& Hopelessness

0   50   100

Problematic   Dangerous

Amount of Sorrow

experiences sorrow, depth of emotion, and a reasonable degree of interiority. Rumi, the mystic poet wrote, "The wound is the place where the Light enters you." This is crucial to the development of empathy, self-reflection, and character formation.

CASE EXAMPLE

Richard, a compilation of various patients who might be located on the lower end of this scale, arrives at the insistence of someone else, perhaps a spouse who insists he seek help. Richard's wife describes him as aloof and distant, unable to relate to her emotions. Richard has been successful in his career but claims few friends. If he has regrets and sorrows, he gives no indication. Richard suffers from a conspicuous lack of introspection, and if he does think about himself and his life, it tends to appear shallow and inconsequential. This lack of capacity for sorrow along with the absence of introspection does not equip Richard to empathize with his children, his wife, or others. Richard has been to marital counseling, but he could never quite grasp that there was anything wrong. For

Richard, life is all right. Upon entering treatment, Richard may acknowledge something must change only because someone else, like a spouse, has made this clear to him. This is not an insight arrived at through his own interior reflection.

Richard's work in therapy may require him to cultivate the capacity to feel sorrow, discontent, and introspection. Richard may never become warm and fuzzy; however, he can develop sufficient tolerance for sorrow and introspection to equip him to empathize with his wife and others.

Of course, it is far more likely that persons located closer to 100 on this scale will present for treatment. These individuals suffer deep depression, characterized by a lack of energy, hopelessness, and despair so profound as to cause them to contemplate suicide. Clinicians will find themselves working diligently to restore such individuals closer to the middle range. Treatment may not achieve such a *Confucian* ideal of the middle way, and it is common for such persons to suffer lingering, *Persistent* depressive symptoms.

CONFUCIAN DOCTRINE OF THE MEAN

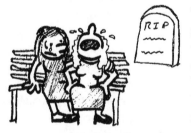

To find oneself in the middle range is optimal. The middle is the domain where we profit from our losses and regrets without becoming overwhelmed by them. From this realm arise empathy, insight, genuine self-regulation, and the fruits of uncovering therapy. This middle range will be fluid in ways that allow a person to descend into the darker realms of human existence while preserving the capacity to emerge again into an engaged, active life. Not only is sorrow and introspection tolerated in the middle region, it is often transmuted into useful results. The middle is where life experience, like the organic material that creates topsoil, is turned, worked, and eventually used as nutrients for soul building. In the middle region, a person does not need to resort to aloof, disengagement nor do they need to fear engulfment by their own despair.

MAJOR DEPRESSIVE DISORDER "SIG E CAPSS" LASTING FOR AT LEAST 2 WEEKS

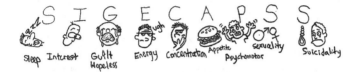

Sleep   Interest   Guilt   Energy   Concentration   Appetite   Psychomotor   Sexuality   Suicidality
Hopeless

Major Depressive Disorder is a very common complaint that leads people to seek treatment. Severe cases of Major Depressive Disorder are challenging to treat. Many clinicians have received the middle-of-the-night call from someone who makes it known they want to take their own life. Depression is one of the deepest forms of human sufferings and suicide or thoughts of suicide is one of its features.

Major Depressive Disorder is established by a number of symptoms that must be present for a sufficient duration. While it technically only requires 2 weeks of symptoms, most patients who present for treatment have suffered for months or years. Treatment typically includes psychotherapy, antidepressant medications, and combinations of both.

PERSISTENT DEPRESSIVE DISORDER

Persistent Depressive Disorder consolidates Major Depression, Recurrent (or chronic) and Dysthymic Disorder. The 12-month prevalence of this disorder is approximately 2%. The causes of Persistent Depressive Disorder are complex, and can include genetic factors, substance abuse, stress, interpersonal issues, endocrinologic factors, childhood issues, trauma, and more. These complex factors make Persistent Depressive Disorder difficult to treat. Treatment inevitably involves several different approaches at once.

PREMENSTRUAL DYSPHORIC DISORDER (PREVIOUSLY PMS)

Some women experience physical and emotional symptoms prior to the onset of menstruation. These symptoms range in severity from mild, barely noticeable changes to severe, disruptive changes. Mood symptoms can include severe mood swings, irritability, anger outbursts, anxiety, and severe depression. Symptoms resolve or substantially improve once menstruation ensues. Women with significant complaints may be diagnosed with *Premenstrual Dysphoric Disorder*. Their lives are shackled to their monthly cycle, and this can be exhausting and exasperating. Treatments for *Premenstrual Dysphoric Disorder* include exercise, diet, antidepressant medication, anti-anxiety medication, hormonal treatment, and psychotherapy.

CONCLUSION

Depressive Disorders are common and produce substantial suffering. Becoming familiar with how to diagnose and treat them is a critically important task for any mental health care provider.

CHAPTER 6

THE MANIA SPECTRUM: BORING VERSUS BIPOLAR

BIPOLAR-WHAT'S NEW IN DSM-5

The core criterion for Bipolar Disorder gives more emphasis to increased energy and increased activity levels than on the qualities of the mood. Just like with Depressive Disorder, the clinician is able to **Specify** the presence of **Mixed Features** where significant depressive symptoms exist and **Anxiety** when there is an anxious component. According to Angst, "a weakness, shown in relation to DSM-IV, was *that it was only able to formally diagnose under half the patients actually treated."*[11]

Boring vs. Bipolar
"How much CREATIVITY do you have?"

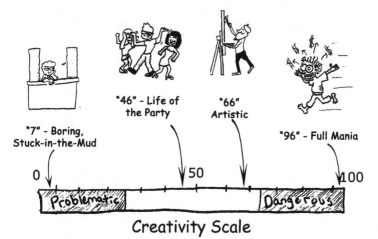

"46" - Life of
the Party

"66"
Artistic

"7" - Boring,
Stuck-in-the-Mud

"96" - Full Mania

0   50   100

Problematic   Dangerous

Creativity Scale

BIPOLAR AS A SPECTRUM OF ILLNESS

In the last decade, Bipolar Disorder received a great deal of attention. There are suggestions that it has become a "trend" to diagnose Bipolar Disorder in virtually all circumstances where mood and affect instability exists. Clinicians may have had the experience of patients who come seeking a diagnosis of Bipolar Disorder. Angst criticized earlier version of the DSM for "…the lack of operationalized subthreshold diagnoses."[12] The rise in the rate of diagnosis differs between adults and youths. According to one study, "While the diagnosis of bipolar disorder in adults increased nearly 2-fold during the 10-year study period, the diagnosis of bipolar disorder in youth increased approximately 40-fold during this period."[13] The reasons for the rise in rates of diagnosis or the reason for the discrepancies between adults and youth are unclear. Perhaps greater media attention combined with the barrage of advertising from pharmaceutical companies that see enormous potential in treating unstable mood and affect are contributors.

Many clinicians may have seen patients presenting with a full complement of bipolar symptoms with discrete episodes of mania and depression. Since severe presentation of mania often leads to hospitalization, many clinicians may seldom see full-blown mania. Muted presentations of Bipolar Disorder are common. Under such circumstances there may be some symptoms that are strongly suggestive of Bipolar Disorder but not clearly established.

In those instances where the diagnosis is unclear, one author tends to rely more heavily upon the presence of a family history of bipolarity while the other author tends to consider "how much" bipolarity a person displays. Both authors have used a *spectrum approach* with Bipolar Disorder for years, recognizing that there is often strong suggestion of *Bipolarity* even in circumstances where all the diagnostic criteria were not met according to earlier versions of the DSM.

The concept of "how much" bipolarity exists can be reassuring, even liberating for many patients. Imagine that all of us exist along a continuum of bipolarity. If we look at the spectrum between "0"

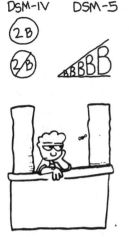

bipolarity and "100" bipolarity, everyone can be placed somewhere along this spectrum. Either extreme of the spectrum typically proves to be problematic.

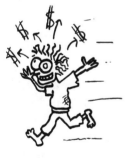

Toward the low end of the spectrum, toward "zero", a person possesses very low energy. Such a person tends to lack creativity, and they can be perceived as boring or flat. Such a person is caricatured as being stuck in an office cubicle, surrounded by stacks of paper, partaking in no creative outlets in their job and perhaps no creative outlets elsewhere. The lack of the quality of *joie de vivre* is obvious. Such a person suffers a global lack of energy and motivation. Their life may appear dull, a chore, lacking spontaneity. This person desperately needs more life force, more *Eros*, more spontaneity.

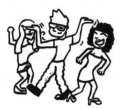

At the other end of the spectrum (toward "100") different problems ensue. Such an individual suffers an overabundance of energy. They cannot slow down, they tend to be overly talkative, they are flooded with many ideas, their thoughts race, and they may experience psychosis with hallucinations. Frequently, they spend too much money and lack restraint. They may give away possessions. Their speech is impulsive and tends to be unfiltered. Someone situated toward "100" on the spectrum will often take risks that others judge to be excessive; they display poor judgment. This person's severe bipolar symptoms need urgent treatment.

Most of us are somewhere in between these 2 extremes. We may tend toward less energy and less spontaneity or we may lean toward higher energy and creativity. Toward the middle of the spectrum there is

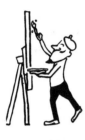 a wide range that encompasses healthy human behavior. The cartoon image in this middle area depicts someone dancing, painting, and enjoying life. He may occasionally be fun, "cool," and the "life of the party". Farther up the scale a person shows signs of gifted artistry. Those at the lower end of the scale might not be the life of the party, but neither are they a black hole of vitality and joy.

"Bipolarity" that remains at sustainable levels, without extremes in either direction may be something of a blessing. A wellspring of creative, artistic energy can be tapped without demonstrating disruptive extremes. This degree of *Bipolarity* is modulated such that a person is equipped to engage life, engage with others, create from nothing, and experience excitement about living. Too much or too little can produce problems for which treatment should be considered.

CLINICAL EXAMPLE

Gloria presented for treatment when things had gone too far. She had always been a fun-loving, gregarious person who enjoyed going out with friends. She worked as an interior designer at a well-known firm where she had been one of the best at her work. When life became more stressful than usual, her sleep worsened. She recounted a series of bad investments, she had become more irritable, and she was becoming more easily distracted. She had become impulsive, and she had been counseled at work about blurting out things that came to her mind. Her spending habits had been out of control for months and her drinking escalated. Gloria had been in a monogamous relationship for several years but recently she had a one-night stand with someone she met while out of town. The straw that broke the camel's back was when she screamed obscenities at her boss, a man she had always admired. While Gloria displayed no psychosis, she certainly had many symptoms along the spectrum of *Bipolarity*. Clearly, her extreme mood was causing problems.

With the help of mood stabilizing medication, something to improve her sleep, and counseling Gloria accepted the idea that treatment would modify and even subdue some of her symptoms without entirely ridding her of all her *Bipolarity*. Instead, a manageable state of creativity and excitement was the goal. Her creativity was honored. As her insomnia, irritability, and impulsivity calmed down, she recovered the ability to "govern" herself and manage her extremes.

In many respects, the criteria for *Bipolar and Related Disorders* in DSM-5 have not changed. Distinctions continue to be made between *Manic Episode, Hypomanic Episode*, and *Major Depressive Episode*. DSM-5 continues to distinguish between *Bipolar Disorder I* and *Bipolar Disorder II*.

CONCLUSION

Bipolar and Related Disorders are common conditions encountered by mental-health practitioners. Discussing *Bipolarity* as a *Spectrum Disorder* can help patients embrace treatment while preserving their dignity and respect. The symptoms of *Bipolar and Related Disorders* present are varied. Even in situations where the boundary between normal creativity and spontaneity and pathology is unclear, the spectrum between *Boring* and *Bipolar* is a useful construct.

CHAPTER 7

THE ANXIETY SPECTRUM: CARELESSNESS VERSUS ANXIOUSNESS

ANXIETY — WHAT'S NEW IN DSM-5

Several diagnoses are no longer found in the Anxiety Disorder section.

Obsessive Compulsive and Related Disorders comprise a **new** category where OCD is to be found.

PTSD has **moved** and is now found under the heading of *Trauma- and Stressor-Related Disorders*. The Anxiety Disorder section has also uncoupled the diagnoses of ***Panic*** and ***Agoraphobia***.

There are 2 diagnoses, *Separation Anxiety Disorder* and *Selective Mutism that* **moved** from the Disorders of Childhood section to the Anxiety Disorder section.

ANXIETY AS A SPECTRUM OF ILLNESS

When considering Anxiety Disorders along a spectrum, the amount of vigilance is the fulcrum on which these phenomenon pivot. The 2 extremes comprise this spectrum, Carelessness versus

Carelessness vs. Anxiousness
"How much VIGILANCE do you have?"

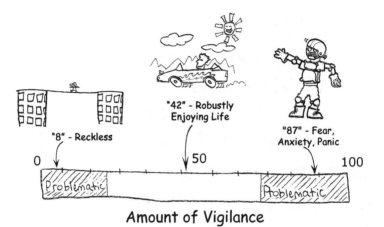

"42" - Robustly
Enjoying Life

"8" - Reckless

"87" - Fear,
Anxiety, Panic

0   50   100

Problematic   Problematic

Amount of Vigilance

Anxiousness. Here the question becomes "how much vigilance do
you have?" The more vigilance a person displays, the more likely
they are to progress to clinical anxiety at some point.

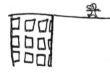

The far left side of the spectrum involves almost no vigilance at all. This
is highly problematic. Such a person
is reckless and lacks the ability to
properly evaluate risk. A certain level
of anxiety is important. Anxiety is a warning system for our body
and mind that something dangerous may be at hand. The capacity
to arouse the autonomic nervous system in order to elicit the *fight
or flight* response is vitally important. According to *Kaplan & Saddock: Concise Guide to Psychiatry:*

> An important aspect of emotions is their effect on the
> selectivity of attention. Anxious persons likely select certain
> things in their environment and overlook others in their effort
> to prove that they are justified in considering the situation
> frightening. If they falsely justify their fear, they augment
> their anxieties by the selective response and set up a vicious

circle of anxiety, distorted perception, and increased anxiety. If, alternatively, they falsely reassure themselves by selective thinking, appropriate anxiety may be reduced, and they may fail to take necessary precautions.[14]

Vigilance is necessary to avoid danger. Depicted in the cartoon at the left side of the scale is a tight-rope walker with no net showing very little vigilance and considerable recklessness.

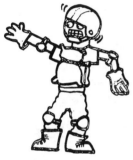

The other end of the spectrum depicts someone possessed of too much vigilance. This person is highly anxious and fearful. The figure is covered with protective gear including a helmet, gloves, boots, kneepads, and even a pillow strapped to his chest to protect him from falls. This is someone who is too cautious, too anxious, and easily overwhelmed with fear. He may well have *Panic Disorder, Generalized Anxiety Disorder* or another anxiety-related illness. Such a high degree of hypervigilance interferes with life.

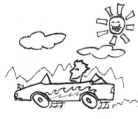

The well-balanced person is depicted as riding down the road in a convertible with the top down. The sun is shining, and though he is driving carefully, his care and caution is not hindering his enjoyment. He balances the risk of driving with the top down with the pleasure of driving a convertible. He has found himself in the sweet spot between appropriate concern or worry and a lack of hypervigilance that would rob life of lightness of being.

PANIC DISORDER

Panic disorder manifests with very intense anxiety that can be terrifying to patients. The initial episode of panic is frequently remembered in vivid detail. Panic Disorder is comprised of discrete episodes of *panic*, and frequently a significant component of *anticipatory anxiety*. During acute bouts of panic, the patient often worries they are having a heart attack or they are going to die. A host of physical symptoms may occur during a panic episode. Patients may present to their physician or to an emergency department for evaluation. After extensive testing that often reveals no clear cause, *Panic Disorder* may be diagnosed by default. This may be the point when referral to a mental health professional occurs. Cognitive behavior psychotherapy combined with low dose antidepressants is a common treatment strategy. Brief courses of anti-anxiety agents, often administered under the tongue for faster onset of action, can help restore a sense of control to patients, but whenever possible caution should be exercised in using anti-anxiety agents like benzodiazepines alone in patients with Panic Disorder.

GENERALIZED ANXIETY DISORDER (GAD)

The person with *GAD* is a worrier. Such persons worry about money, health, stress, work, home, play, and anything else they can imagine. Physical symptoms such as tension, fatigue, poor concentration, insomnia, and irritability frequently accompany their chronic worrying and anxiety. While it appears less acute and less overwhelming than panic disorder, *GAD* produces considerable distress. Treatment may involve psychotherapy, biofeedback, antidepressant medications, beta-blockers, and occasional sparing use of sedatives.

SOCIAL PHOBIA

The lifetime prevalence of Social Phobia is approximately 3%. It seems to occur in people who are also shy and introverted. Sufferers hate being in the spotlight or drawing attention to themselves. Interacting with strangers can be exquisitely painful. Their numerous anxieties cause the person who suffers Social Phobia to avoid situations that make them anxious. This disorder can be debilitating, and sufferers often limit their social, educational, and career opportunities as a consequence of their pervasive anxiety. Treatment involves psychotherapy, skills training, antidepressants, and occasionally sedatives. Validation of the specific features of Social Phobia goes a long way to easing the alienation felt by its sufferers.

SPECIFIC PHOBIA

Specific phobias include a broad range of fears that arise in relation to a specific stimulus. Common phobias include fear of heights, fear of snakes, and fear of spiders. Because the provocation can be very circumscribed, avoidance is more likely to prove effective. When exposure to the stimulus cannot be avoided or if the symptoms severely interfere, patients may seek treatment. Cognitive Behavior Therapy can be very helpful in reducing specific fears. Systematic desensitization as well as flooding techniques can prove helpful.

CONCLUSION

Anxiety symptoms are very common in the general population. They are frequently seen in combination with other illnesses such as Major Depressive Disorder. Anxiety has adaptive and maladaptive aspects. One way of conceptualizing Anxiety Disorders is to imagine the symptoms pivoting around an axis of vigilance.

CHAPTER 8

THE PSYCHOSIS SPECTRUM: VISIONLESS VERSUS PSYCHOTIC

WHAT'S NEW IN DSM-5

The 5 subtypes of Schizophrenia have been eliminated (catatonic, disorganized, paranoid, residual, and undifferentiated). Catatonia, however, is still used as a Specifier that can be employed with Schizophrenia, Bipolar Disorder or Depression. The diagnoses of schizophrenia must now include at least 1 positive symptom—hallucinations, delusions, or disorganized speech.

With Schizoaffective disorder, either depression or bipolarity must be present for a majority of the disorder's total duration.

PSYCHOSIS AS A SPECTRUM OF ILLNESS

Of the *8 Primary Spectrums of Psychiatry* described in this book that exist along a continuum between normal functioning and illness, psychosis is the hardest one in which to identify a range of normal expression. However, the more one considers the psychoses the more one can recognize certain healthy elements within the milder aspects of the psychosis spectrum. If we change "how psychotic are you?" to "how strong are your dreams and visions?" a spectrum begins to emerge for the cluster of symptoms common to psychosis. Almost everyone has some level of inspiring dreams or visions or meaningful experiences. We may awaken in the middle of the night convinced that something has happened and be surprised to realize it was "just a dream." For those few minutes we are out of touch with reality and still possessed by the dream. We might also have a breakthrough, an unusually inspiring thought or idea. It might seem to come from outside oneself. Many people have heard voices, seen things that others did not see, or experienced moments of precognition. Strictly speaking these may be considered hallucinations or delusions. They can also be considered as eruptions from other part of the psyche, perhaps even beyond the psyche. Poets, authors, and artists sometimes describe "being a channel for the art trying to incarnate itself." They claim that they didn't produce it themselves, but just let it come out through them. Others will have powerful spiritual experiences. They may see a vision of a deceased relative, hear their voice briefly or even hear God speak to them at times. This is most often not formal psychosis, but rather normal human experience of the divine or the normal grieving process of having lost a loved one. These experiences, however, are all on the spectrum of various intensities of dreams and visions. If these dreams and visions become intense and overwhelming enough, then the border between real and unreal starts to break down. The vision becomes a persistent hallucination or the "voice of God" becomes delusional in its intensity or bizarreness. Thus, even psychosis can have a range of normal human expression.

Visionless vs. Psychotic:
"How strong are your DREAMS and VISIONS?"

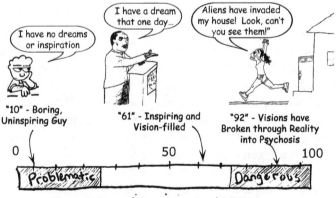

Intensity of Dreams and Visions

Our illustration is titled "Visionless vs. Psychotic: how strong are your dreams and visions?" The scale on the bottom indicates the strength of theses dreams and visions. As usual, either end of the spectrum is problematic and trying to hold the middle is the optimal result.

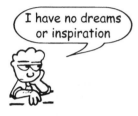

On the left end of the spectrum is an individual with no dreams or inspirations. He is a boring sort of a guy with little spontaneity or future goals. It's hard for him to imagine his life in the future since his imagination is so limited. He had trouble playing any games as a child that required thinking outside the box, role-playing, or other imaginal pieces. When he tried to draw a picture, his mind stayed empty and the paper stayed blank. He dislikes art, drama, or even theoretical physics in college; they required too much imagination. Spirituality has little meaning for him, as he cannot see anything beyond the physical reality of the here and now. He cannot remember any of his dreams and does not experience inspiring thoughts. He has a hard time making choices like a career path or even where to live, because he is devoid of vision for the future. While such a person doesn't always come in for treatment, this individual deeply needs the help of a skilled psychotherapist or spiritual director to get him out of this dry, lifeless space.

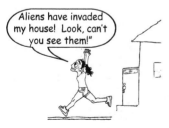

The person on the right has a different and more serious problem. She is being flooded by the dream world and is no longer in touch with reality. She has lost the filter that most of us possess that allows us to know the difference between what is real and what is fantasy. She is full of delusions and she has become convinced that aliens invaded our planet and are taking over her neighborhood. She has visual hallucination, seeing images of these aliens attacking. She further believes they have been monitoring her phone and spying on her actions. She hears voices incessantly. The voices give her instructions, as if they direct her thoughts and actions. They are sometimes dark and critical and occasionally tell her to give up. It is absolutely terrifying to develop psychotic symptoms of this intensity. It is arguably the worst of our psychiatric diagnoses. She is in urgent need of hospitalization, antipsychotic medications, and acute stabilization.

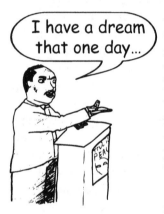

As always, the middle region of this spectrum is the optimal realm. This is where the soul thrives and where we can reach our highest potential. It is the land of the visionaries that we all admire or strive to become and where occasionally we all dwell. It is the domain that gives rise to people like Martin Luther King Jr., Mother Teresa, Mahatma Gandhi, John F. Kennedy, and countless others who inspire us. People living in the middle of this spectrum are full of inspirations, hopes, and dreams.

Most people have visionary moments in their life in which we are swept up in something larger than ourselves. Perhaps we awaken in the middle of the night awestruck with a new idea and the possibilities it offers. On such occasions we have entered the middle region between boring and psychotic. Such moments need not be grand, sometimes they may involve the solution to a vexing problem or the unexpected reminder of a special occasion of a loved one that warrants acknowledgement. Any powerful new idea, goal, vision, or hope is in this territory. Whereas psychosis can be a terrifying experience that threatens to rupture the very vessel of psychological container, experiences arising in the middle region of this spectrum can be profound and transformative, catalyzing enormous change. At times, the experience of being comfortably in this middle region is rich, meaningful, and even sacramental. Life is neither bland nor excessively spicy; it has the right seasoning to bring out the best flavor.

DIAGNOSES IN DETAIL

SCHIZOPHRENIA

Schizophrenia involves losing touch with reality. It often includes hallucinations that are defined by a perception without an associated stimulus. They include auditory, visual, tactile, and/or olfactory hallucinations. Persons with schizophrenia can be disorganized and act in highly unusual ways. Delusions, defined as fixed, false beliefs, are often present and can be bizarre at times.

SCHIZOAFFECTIVE DISORDER

Schizoaffective disorder is best thought of as a mixture of symptoms and signs that are associated with Schizophrenia and mood disorders (bipolar or depression). Individuals with schizoaffective disorder must have evidence of a major mood disorder present the majority of the time that they are symptomatic. Like schizophrenia, this disorder can be debilitating.

Delusional disorder is characterized by a well-circumscribed delusion in the context of otherwise well preserved functioning.

CONCLUSION

Psychosis viewed along a spectrum spans a terrifying realm of human experience as well as the realm from which inspiration and visionary ideas arise. The clinician is advised to remember that there is often a fine line that separates madness and genius. The middle region of the Psychosis spectrum is fertile and inspired. It does not lead others to immediately conclude that a person is insane. By viewing psychosis along a spectrum from thoroughly boring and uninspired to fully overtaken by visions and delusions, the clinician can navigate the inner landscape with a proper balance of respect, caution, and inspiration of their own.

CHAPTER 9

THE FOCUS SPECTRUM: ATTENTION DEFICIT DISORDER VERSUS OBSESSIVE COMPULSIVE AND RELATED DISORDERS

ADHD AND OCD—WHAT'S NEW IN DSM-5

DSM-5 has added a new group of disorders known as the *Obsessive Compulsive and Related Disorders*. This category includes *OCD*, *Body Dysmorphic Disorder*, and *Trichotillomania*.

There are newly created diagnoses in this section that include *Hoarding Disorder* and *Excoriation (skin picking) Disorder*.

Attention Deficit Hyperactivity Disorder (ADHD) has remained virtually unchanged.

ADHD AND OCD AS A SPECTRUM OF ILLNESS

The spectrum proposed here combines 2 categories in DSM-5 that can be related to one another by the degree of focus a person maintains. Strictly speaking OCD's ancestral roots link it to anxiety disorders and not ADHD. However, these 2 disorders move about an axis that is related to how much capacity for focused attention the patient displays. Someone with very little focus might be suffering *Attention Deficit Hyperactivity Disorder*, while somebody with extreme focus, perhaps even an inability to change their focus of attention from a ruminative thought might be diagnosed with *OCD*.

Attention Deficit Disorder (ADHD) vs. Obsessive Compulsive Disorder (OCD) "How much FOCUS do you have?"

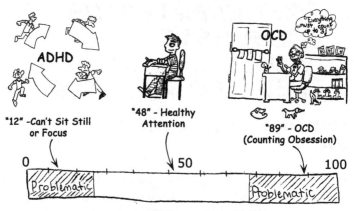

Amount of Focusing Ability

In our illustration we have labeled the primary variable as the amount of focusing someone has.

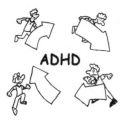

The far left of the diagram depicts a person with almost no focusing ability. This person cannot maintain focus on a single task for very long. Their mind wanders; they are very distractible and jump from project to project. This person likely has ADHD.

Equally problematic is the other end of the spectrum on the right side of the diagram. This person has too much focus. They are unable to shift their focus of attention and often go over the same detail or worry repeatedly. Persons with OCD become locked into obsessive patterns of thinking. These patterns may include:

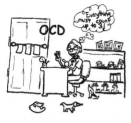

counting rituals, hand-washing, excessive orderliness, a need for symmetry, germ phobias, and myriad other obsessions. The consequences of such ceaseless obsessions, compulsions, and rituals range from mild annoyance to significant impairment in work and social life. Severely afflicted individuals may seem to be enslaved by their obsessive compulsive rituals and routines. Treatment often consists of medications (most commonly SSRIs) and behavioral treatment.

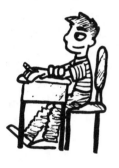

The middle part of the diagram depicts the Spectrum of Focus. A person is shown whose degree of focus is properly balanced. Such an individual can pay attention for extended periods of time, for example, in a lecture. Their ability to maintain their focus of attention still allows for flexible shifts in attention. They are not imprisoned by their attention like someone with OCD, but can flexibly allow their thoughts and actions to shift from one focus to another. A person located in the middle region of this spectrum will not drift aimlessly or haphazardly from one topic to another, nor will they gravitate to every shiny new object they encounter like the person with ADHD. Individuals with ADHD have difficulty sustaining attention when something is no longer of high interest to them. The ideal or goal with regard to the Focus Spectrum is to strike an effective balance between well-focused attention and shifting focus of attention. This is the middle ground. Straying to either extreme end of the spectrum proves problematic and requires *professional* attention.

CLINICAL EXAMPLE

Pete is a patient whose focus places him at the extreme end. He has always been an orderly and high-achieving man. As a child, Pete kept his room neat and clean, he turned in his homework on time after checking it over numerous times, and he often felt anxious that he might have done something wrong that would come back to haunt him. He excelled in school and was well-liked. Pete's tendencies and idiosyncrasies intensified when he reached high school. He would become terribly upset and anxious if his homework was not exactly right and this required him to spend long hours completing assignments, longer than others thought necessary. His morning routine to get ready for school took progressively longer as he added more rituals and routines that had to be performed exactly the same way and in the same order each day. Upon graduation from high school Pete took a job overseeing quality control at a local factory. His relentless attention to detail garnered favorable attention at work though many coworkers, who found his perfectionism unbearable, disliked him. He kept both his home and workplace spotlessly clean. When he began to feel that there were germs on various surfaces, he started using Clorox cleaning sheets on his phone, keyboard, countertops, and certain personal belongings. By the time he sought treatment he reported cleaning the kitchen 4 times each day, he had rituals that governed how dishes should be stacked, and he was insistent that toilet paper rolls be hung a certain way. Pete's friends poked fun at him for his overly focused attention by sometimes leaving small pieces of trash on the floor to see how long it would take him to notice and clean it up.

A year before he sought treatment Pete's mother was diagnosed with emphysema that required her to rely on continuous oxygen. One day the idea popped into his head that she might run out of oxygen so he began calling her 5 times a day to make sure her breathing was alright. He found it hard to fall asleep as he began to worry before bed about her health. His focus on germs increased and he began washing his hands every 20 or 30 minutes. His hands became red and excoriated. He developed slightly magical beliefs in which he grew convinced that if he did not pray in a certain manner and at certain times, God would not hear his prayers. If he messed up one word in the prayer, he felt compelled to start from the beginning and pray again. The numerous things he felt the need to focus upon consumed more time and Pete began to withdraw from people.

He was referred for treatment when his hand washing resulted in severe dermatitis and he was diagnosed with *OCD*, started on an SSRI (sertraline), and referred for cognitive behavioral therapy. The medicine helped Pete loosen his focus of attention on the things that now were plaguing him and therapy furthered the goal of subduing his exaggerated focus of attention. Pete learned to redirect his focus of attention away from obsessive ruminations and with the help of the medicine he found he could free himself from the endless loops and eddies of thought he had known his entire life. Pete was pleased to discover that medicine and therapy did nothing to loosen his careful attention to detail at work, but he no longer felt compelled to correct coworker's every mistake, just the ones that affected quality control.

DIAGNOSES IN DETAIL

OBSESSIVE COMPULSIVE DISORDER AND RELATED DISORDERS

The OCDs are distinct from ADHD in DSM-5 and clinicians are encouraged to keep in mind that the Focus Spectrum provides a model for understanding and is not intended to conflate ADHD and OCD.

OCD and related disorders have in common an excessive degree of focus. These disorders include:

Obsessive Compulsive Disorder (OCD) This is characterized by *Obsessions* that consist of persistent, intrusive, unwanted thoughts, urges, or images and *Compulsions* that are repetitive behaviors intended to suppress or neutralize obsessions with other thoughts or actions. Both obsessions and compulsions are time consuming and distressing.

Common symptoms include rituals involving checking, counting, cleaning, and the need for symmetry. Sufferers may have fears of losing control or they may worry incessantly that they will engage in forbidden actions. Clinicians can specify the degree of insight (with good or fair insight, with poor insight, with absent insight/delusional beliefs). There is also a Tic-related Specifier available. Even those with insight are unable to fend off their OCD symptoms. Treatment may include medications and cognitive behavioral psychotherapy. Medications are most often serotonergic antidepressants, usually at higher dosages.

Body Dysmorphic Disorder
• Specify: with muscle dysmorphia, and with good/fair insight, poor insight, absent insight/delusional beliefs.

Body Dysmorphic Disorder can be a very challenging illness to treat. Patients become utterly convinced that they have a severe body defect, usually cosmetic in nature. Even if there is a slight defect, their obsession about this small defect is much greater than is warranted. They focus on their perceived defect. They may consult plastic surgeons who hesitate to operate when their perceived defect is not detectable or objectively verified.[15] At some point in the disorder sufferers will have engaged in repetitive or checking behavior. There are several specifiers including with muscle dysmorphia, and with good/fair insight, poor insight, absent insight/delusional beliefs. Medications can help slightly, but often response is marginal. Psychotherapy is the most effective course.

Trichotillomania   Presents with recurrent hair pulling resulting in hair loss. There is a cycle of tension (when hair pulling is resisted) and relief (when hair pulling ensues). These features produce significant distress and impairment.

Hoarding Disorder   With muscle dysmorphia, and with good/fair insight, poor insight, absent insight/delusional beliefs. A hallmark of this disorder is the inability to discard possessions, regardless of the value. Sufferers perceive the need to save things and become distressed with having to discard items. The person with Hoarding Disorder suffers distress and impairment.

Excoriation (skin picking) Disorder.   This disorder manifests with skin picking that results in lesions or skin infections. The common features of tension and relief found in trichotillomania and the element of distress and impairment are characteristic.

Attention-Deficit Hyperactivity Disorder (ADHD)   There are 2 broad characteristics of ADHD, Inattention and Hyperactivity/impulsivity. The disorder results in social, occupational, or school impairment. The different types are listed below.

Attention Deficit Hyperactivity Disorder (ADHD) is usually diagnosed in childhood. School-aged children may demonstrate difficulty in the classroom from either the inattention and/or hyperactivity. Work may be left unfinished, homework may not be turned in, disruptive behavior may occur in the classroom. The hyperactive components may include restlessness, fidgetiness, calling out in class, and other inappropriate behavior. While ADHD may improve by adulthood, the symptoms often persist causing difficulties in work and personal life.[16][17][18][19] A multimodal treatment that includes behavior modification, medications, or combinations of the 2 is common.[20] Various medications are used including stimulants (amphetamine and amphetamine-like molecules), antidepressants, Atomoxetine (*Strattera*, a nonstimulant, Norepinephrine reuptake inhibitor), antihypertensive agents (adrenergic agonists like Clonidine, *Catapres,* or guanfacine hydrochloride, *Tenex.* Close coordination with teachers and education of families is important.

CONCLUSION

Although DSM-5 does not link ADHD and OCD and Related Disorders, a common thread courses through them both. The amount of focus a person displays can be a defining feature of where a person lies on this spectrum. For persons at the left end of this spectrum (ADHD), treatment strives to increase their ability to maintain focus. For persons at the right end of the spectrum (OCD) the goal is to temper their excessive focus of attention.

CHAPTER 10

THE SUBSTANCE ABUSE SPECTRUM: ASCETIC VERSUS ADDICTED

At first we liv'd in pleasure;
Thine own delights thou didst to us impart;
When we grew wanton, thou didst use displeasure
To make us thine: ...
(Excerpt from *Afflcitions* by George Herbert)

SUBSTANCE-RELATED AND ADDICTIVE DISORDERS— WHAT'S NEW IN DSM-5

There are several changes in DSM-5 pertaining to substance abuse.

 Gambling Disorder is now recognized as sharing such common features with substance abuse disorders that it has been moved to this category. One big change is that DSM-5 no longer distinguishes between *substance abuse* and *substance dependence*. DSM-5 adopts a "spectrum" approach. *Substance-related and Addictive Disorders* encompass *Alcohol-related Disorder, Cannabis-related Disorder, Opioid-related Disorder*, etc.). *Tobacco-related Disorder* has also been added to the list of substance of abuse. Within each *Substance-related Disorder* exists a spectrum of severity described as *mild, moderate,* or *severe*. The severity correlates with the number of criteria met by a person. Each substance of abuse can be further delineated establishing whether or not the person is *intoxicated* or *withdrawing.*

SUBSTANCE ABUSE AS A SPECTRUM OF ILLNESS

Another of the *8 Primary Spectrums of Mental Illness* is substance abuse. The global burden of substance abuse is enormous and in the United States the burden of tobacco, alcohol, and illicit drugs exceeds $600 billion annually.[21] Substance-related and Addictive Disorders are a common primary diagnosis and are frequently a comorbid diagnosis. Clinicians cannot escape the importance of understanding substance abuse and its treatment. *Alcoholics Anonymous, Celebrate Recovery,* and other 12-step recovery groups are mainstays of treatment for many people. Treatment options include a wide array of options such as inpatient confinement, long-term residential treatment, outpatient programs, individual therapy, and pharmacologic interventions. Pharmacologic interventions may include *methadone, Suboxone, Campral, Bupropion, and traditional psychiatric medication.*

Certain ideas and words arising from the domain of addiction and its treatment have found their way into our lexicon. It is common to hear about various "addictions" like *sexual addictions, shopping addictions, nicotine addictions, caffeine addictions, workaholism, and Internet addictions.* Two of these involve a psychoactive compound that affects CNS receptors. The others rely upon the common denominator of **craving** that addictive phenomena share. None of these are recognized in DSM-5. Many other words such as *codependency, dysfunctional, denial, dry drunk* have entered common usage. By extending the principles from the realm of addiction and recovery we see that virtually any activity that brings pleasure and involves intense craving can be misused in an addictive manner.

When viewed through the lens of "pleasure-seeking behavior" and immediate gratification, Substance-related and Addictive Disorders share a great deal in common regardless of the substance or behavior involved. There is a spectrum ranging from the ascetic to the person who chronically yields to pleasure-seeking and craving. The middle region of this spectrum is epitomized in the old adage, "All things in moderation." The caricatures depicted in the cartoons at the extreme are an "ascetic monk" and a "party animal" with raging addictions. In Analytical (Jungian) psychology, disavowing a psychic element and relegating it to the shadow increases the likelihood of being overtaken or blindsided by it. We recall examples of evangelists and politicians who publicly rebuke sexual immorality only to be caught in the very same acts they denounce. From a Jungian perspective the middle region of this spectrum is achieved via the *transcendent function* that fosters a *conjunctio* or conjunction of opposites.

Ascetic Monk vs. Multiple Addictions: "How Much PLEASURE Do You Seek?"

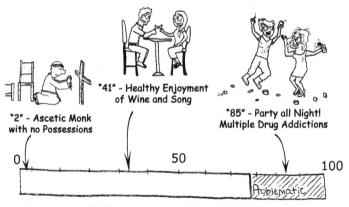

Amount of Pleasure Seeking / Addictiveness

St. Augstine   St. Augstine the youth
Madame Bovary constrained   Madame Bovary in passion

The spectrum of Substance-Related and Addictive Disorder is titled "Ascetic Monk vs. Multiple Addictions: How Much Pleasure Do You Seek?" The feature being assessed that determines where a person is on the spectrum involves the intensity of craving, the pull upon a person that pleasure-seeking behavior exerts. It also involves whether a person overregulates their pleasure-seeking behavior or overindulges their desires.

On the left side of the scale, the ascetic monk either lacks motivation and a desire for pleasure or has so thoroughly restrained himself that the flames of passions are nearly extinguished. Such an ascetic lives simply, perhaps with few belongings. He is careful not to allow too much excitement to inflame him. Such a person may be virtually celibate, they are austere, obedient, and abide by Spartan rules. The material world and its pleasures do not hold sway in his life. Such a lifestyle befits an actual monk but otherwise it presents a problem. If this individual seeks treatment at all, they may need to surrender to pleasures and delights, loosen up, and have fun. Such persons seem incapable of enjoyment, not because they are depressed and anhedonic, but because pleasure-seeking is too tightly governed.

Consider, Maria, the novitiate in *The Sound of Music.* Her natural, irrepressibly joyful temperament was constrained in the monastic life. In fact, once Maria deals with her own excessive asceticism by becoming the children's nanny, she takes on the project of dismantling Captain von Trapp's regimented household that is Spartan-like. The movie is an example of the tension between asceticism and indulgence. When love springs forth and Maria is confronted by the Mother Superior she realizes that she has been hiding in the convent. She and Captain von Trapp are free to explore the vast middle region where pleasure dwells but not in such excess that it enslaves a person.

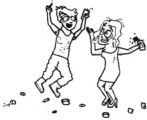 On the far right of the spectrum is a person who might be described as a **party animal**. This person is almost entirely motivated by seeking pleasure. They rarely deny themselves anything. Rather, they are always reaching for the next thrill or another exciting experience. The ordinary life can be painful or distressing to them so they often take risks in order to feel excitement, pleasure, and relief. The relief they seek leads to hazards and such a person is at high risk for addiction, often multiple ad-

dictions. They may get one addiction under control only to have another one spring up. In the thirst for pleasure and relief from distress this person may become dependent on alcohol, pain medications, drugs of abuse (cocaine, ecstasy, LSD, etc), pornography, sex, tobacco, shopping, and a nearly endless list of other things associated with **craving** for pleasure. Denial is an integral part of the addictive disorders and sufferers seldom acknowledge that they have a problem. Eventually, when their *house of cards* collapses as a consequence of their addictions, they may be driven into some form of treatment. Maybe their spouse grows weary and is fed up, or another in a series of job losses occurs, or they run afoul of the law. A popular idea in **12-Step Recovery** circles is that a person must "hit rock bottom" before they are likely to admit they are **powerless** and that their **life** has become **unmanageable.** Only then does the long road to recovery begin in earnest. Treatment often includes participation in a 12-Step recovery group, individual therapy, and in some instances a period of confinement in a substance abuse rehabilitation program. Medications are used judiciously in people with addictions. Research concerning addiction offers promising possibilities for future treatments.[22]

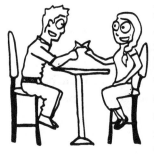

Like with all other *Spectrums of Mental Illness,* the optimal place to be on this scale that assesses pleasure-seeking behavior is in the middle region. In that region, life is enjoyed, pleasure is sought, and the material world can be appreciated. Occasional splurges and moments of decadence are neither entirely absent nor do they dominate the background of a person's life. An occasional drink, a glass of wine, or a beer may be consumed, but those prone to addictions or who have addicted family members may be wise to exercise caution. In the middle, a person may drink without throwing caution to the wind by driving; they recognize risks and avoid them. There is a growing recognition that living in the present moment has many benefits. Whether we call it *mindfulness, The Power of Now, carpe diem (seize the day), radical acceptance, practicing presence, seren-*

ity, or contemplative living, all these approaches share in common a surrender to living in the moment. For the addicted person, such strategies may not be associated with the wildest excitement but there can be rich, vibrant experiences free of hazard that rivals the wild days of addiction. For the ascetic there is such extreme denial and abnegation that their life becomes little more than an ellipsis between their first and last breath.

CONCLUSION

Sadly, Substance-related and Addictive Disorders are common. Addiction does not respect any ethnic, sociocultural, religious, racial, or other boundaries. These disorders are often recalcitrant, and treatment may have to occur several times before success is achieved. In 12-Step recovery groups there exists a belief that addiction usually leads either to death or incarceration. Too often, that proves true. This chapter goes beyond the formulaic approach of DSM-IV where diagnosis implied assessing whether or not a person met criteria for the disorder. With the arrival of DSM-5, the clinician is encouraged to approach Substance-related and Addictive Disorders as phenomenon that exist along a spectrum. In addition, the particular substance of abuse, while noted, appears less central to conceptualizing these disorders than the shared features of craving, high risk tolerance, and social impairment. On the scale presented in this chapter, each of us falls somewhere between the person cut off from all sensual pleasures and the person whose insatiable craving runs the show.

CHAPTER 11

THE AUTISM SPECTRUM: CODEPENDENT VERSUS AUTISTIC

AUTISM—WHAT'S NEW IN DSM-5

DSM-5 has combined *Autism, Asperger's, Childhood Disintegrative Disorder* and *Pervasive Developmental Disorder NOS* into 1 diagnostic category known as *Autism Spectrum Disorder (ASD)*. These diagnoses are now grouped under the broad heading of *Neurodevelopmental Disorders.* Considerable controversy and fear was stirred by the changes introduced to these disorders with DSM-5 and their implications. For instance, *Asperger's Syndrome,* a diagnosis that may have carried less stigma than Autism, is now subsumed by a diagnosis using the term *autism.* **ASD** is characterized by 1) deficits in social communication and social interaction and 2) restricted repetitive behaviors. If only social communication and interaction is impaired, then *Social Communication Disorder* is diagnosed.

AUTISM AS A SPECTRUM OF ILLNESS

Added to the fact that ASD uses the word *spectrum* in its name, the popularization of the *Asperger's Syndrome* contributed to the decision to include Autism as one of the *8 Primary Spectrums of Mental Illness.* When a diagnosis enters the lexicon to such an extent that Asperger's is tossed about as an adjective, it suggests the concept has captured something that was widely understood if not previously named. To say someone is *Asperger's* is not always synonymous with a formal diagnosis. Instead, it may imply that the subject's social skills are askew and that his or her capacity to interpret the social cues most of us take for granted, is impaired. Ironically, just as the concept of a spectrum of Autism and Asperger's has found its way into common usage, the DSM-5 removed *Asperger's* as a diagnosis. Concern has erupted over whether these changes will restrict or expand eligibility for services for children with ASD.

The scale used to illustrate this *Primary Spectrum of Mental Illness* depends upon the clinician assessing the degree to which a person is interpersonally connected, or "how connected to others are you?" The range described spans individuals who are too connected and those who are nearly completely unconnected. The choice of *un*-connected instead of *dis*-connected reflects an appreciation for the fact that to become disconnected, one must first connect. Individuals with *ASD* typically struggle to connect in the first place.

Autism vs. Codependency:
How CONNECTED to Others are you?

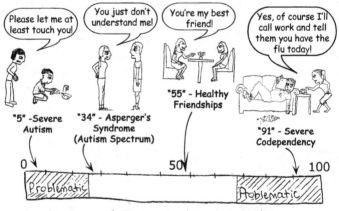

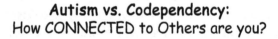

Degree of Connectedness to Others

On the far right end of the spectrum appear people who seem overly connected to others. They are people who become *enmeshed* and whose boundaries are too porous when it comes to the emo-

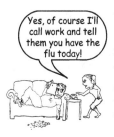

tional stuff of people around them. The term *Codependency* is used for the spectrum though it is strictly speaking, a misapplication of the term. *Codependency* within the recovery movement pertains to the patterns in relationship with an addict or alcoholic wherein a person becomes "addicted" to managing the unmanageable behavior and consequences of their addicted partner. Whereas the addict is dependent upon a substance, the *codependent* person is dependent upon managing the addict. Nevertheless, the spectrum proposed here borrows the term *Codependency* because it aptly fits the sort of excessive and unhealthy connection that is meant.

In addition to the *enmeshed, Codependent* quality that an individual at the extreme right side of scale displays, they sometimes cannot tolerate being alone. They are overinvolved in others' lives. They frequently "need to be needed," and they have difficulty when people in their circle exert independence from them. This may present special problems for their children as they reach developmental stages when autonomy surges. The connected person may gravitate toward people who lack the ability to manage their own lives effectively and who lack self-governance. In this respect, the term *Codependence* captures the idea.

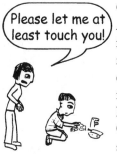

On the left end of the scale is the territory of ASD. The cartoon depicts the most extreme form of *Autism* where even the most minimal interaction with others, like touch, can be experienced as disruptive. This person's difficulties in relationship began in early childhood; they did not relate like other children. Children with severe disorders often come to attention early and are seldom missed. They barely communicate, they engage in repetitive behaviors. Early intervention often includes intensive therapy, medication to manage behavior, and case management services. Diagnosis of children with less severe conditions may be delayed.

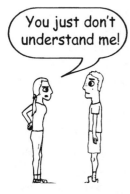

Toward the middle region, but still in a range where problems ensue, the person depicted would have been diagnosed with *Asperger's Syndrome* using DSM-IV. The man's wife is exasperated by his utter lack of comprehension about the simplest sorts of things that most human beings understand. She is calling out to her husband "You just don't understand me!" She is correct because the person with *Asperger's Syndrome* does not decipher ordinary social cues. When he does, it is often because he has learned a set of rules by rote memory that he applies in a stilted, predetermined fashion. He is a successful software engineer, in part, because he likes the logic that governs writing computer code. He trained to be an audiologist because the engineering and technology involved with testing equipment and amplification devices fascinated him. In fact, years after leaving that profession because he found the high demand for human interaction intolerable, he is still able to recite technical specifications of certain hearing aids from memory. His only friends were developed in high school, and they have always made allowances for him. Many people mistake his robotic manner for a lack of feeling and empathy, when in fact it is simply a feature of his poor ability to read social cues (his own and others').

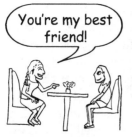

As always, the middle ground is the goal. Here we see 2 women enjoying lunch together. One exclaims that the other is her "best friend." There is the feeling of mutual friendship. Their care for one another is best described as *interdependent*. Individuals in the middle display the quality described by the Buddhist teacher, Thich Nhat Hanh as *Inter-being*. This word, *Inter-being*, connotes a compassionate interconnectedness between all things. Such connectedness is vital, responsive, and meaningful without the pitfalls of enmeshment, codependence, or overbearing control of the other people.

CLINICAL EXAMPLE

Amanda was an oncology nurse whose life centered upon her only child. She presented for treatment 2 months after her son left for college. During her son's senior year of high school, she left her job doing direct patient care in hopes of enjoying more time at home with her son during his senior year of high school. Her husband worked in sales and drank excessively. Under the guise of wining and dining his clients, Amanda's husband tried to cover up his drinking. Amanda was endlessly picking up the slack for her husband. A month before their son left for college, her husband was charged with a DUI. He quit drinking and began attending AA meetings. Instead of late night business meetings, he began attending AA meeting every day of the week. When he would return from a meeting he retired to his workshop where he disappeared for hours at a time. When he began to use AA to begin really attending to the demands of his home life, Amanda grew increasingly distressed and began to complain of feeling useless. She complained of feeling depressed and spoke of feeling anxious that she would end up all alone, with nobody to care for, no child, no husband, and no patients who needed her. For more than 3 months she had not had to rush out of the house late at night to pick up her husband after receiving a call from a concerned client of his. It had been 3 months since she made a call to her husband's employer to cover for him. She began to experience insomnia, crying spells, and pervasive anxiety. Amanda was on the far right end of the scale where *codependency, enmeshed care taking, and overly nurturing* behavior is rampant. She was prescribed an antidepressant, but more importantly, she entered therapy where she dealt with her overly connected, enmeshed style of relating. She started attending *Al-Anon* and the tools she acquired there proved invaluable in subduing a lifetime of codependent behavior; she thrived.

The extreme end of the scale is not described. It suffices to mention that profound (*pervasive*) impairment of communication and repetitive behaviors are common features of this extreme end of the spectrum.

CONCLUSION

This chapter presents a scale to illustrate one of the *8 Primary Spectrums of Mental Illness* based on the degree of connectedness a person displays. Along this scale from *Autism* to *Codependence* the pivotal question is "how connected are you?" Too much connectedness results in states of overenmeshment and codependency where a person's ability to maintain appropriate boundaries is impaired or underdeveloped. At the other extreme of connectedness, individuals are unable to connect with others. The optimal region in the middle demonstrates a capacity for connection and interdependence that does not manifest in excessive connectedness or enmeshment. The word *inter-being* is a good way of characterizing the middle region of this spectrum.

CHAPTER 12

THE PERSONALITY SPECTRUM: NEUROTIC VERSUS OBNOXIOUS

PERSONALITY DISORDERS—WHAT'S NEW IN DSM-5

The most drastic revision concerning personality disorders in DSM-5 is the elimination of the multi-axial diagnostic system. **The multi-axial diagnostic system is abolished.** Therefore, personality disorder diagnoses appear just like any other diagnosis but the disorders themselves were not eliminated. The criteria for personality disorders are almost unchanged in DSM-5. *Antisocial Personality Disorder* also appears under the heading of *Disruptive, Impulse-Control, and Conduct Disorders*. This makes sense since most clinicians understand *Conduct Disorder* and *Oppositional Defiant Disorder* to be the predecessor of *Antisocial Personality Disorder*. All 10 personality disorders from DSM-IV are carried over into DSM-5.

PERSONALITY DISORDERS AS A SPECTRUM OF ILLNESS

The concept of personality fits very well into the conceptual framework of illness along a spectrum. The scale for personality disorders, another of the *8 Primary Spectrums of Mental Illness,* encompasses all 10 disorders. A **fundamental feature** of personality disorders is the tendency people with these disorders have to ***externalize* blame** or causation for their symptoms.

Individuals who suffer personality disorder have problems conducting the daily affairs of their lives and often have problems relating to others. When something goes wrong, they immediately locate the source of their problems outside of themselves (this can also be described as having an ***external locus of control***).[23] In contrast, the right side of the scale depicts individuals who an earlier version of the DSM (II) described as *neurotic*. At the extreme left end of the scale, the *neurotic* end, individuals ascribe exaggerated and excessive cause or blame to themselves for anything that goes wrong.

People with personality disorders are also characterized by **rigidity** and **inflexibility** in the way they live and the way they relate to others. They do not learn from their experience and they do not change; they do not adapt. Repeated experiences that should demonstrate to the sufferer that they have a role in their own struggles fail to inform them. Instead, when a pattern of problems repeats they interpret it as further evidence that others are to blame for their difficulties. This is the meaning of *maladaptive*. Clinicians may find such patient's defenses to be almost impenetrable. It can prove helpful to keep in mind that their inability to recognize their own role in their problems and the turmoil that surrounds them is a pivotal feature.

A certain amount of quirkiness and idiosyncrasy is to be expected across the range of normal human personality function. However, personality disordered individuals display an exaggerated amount of idiosyncratic thought, perception, and behavior. If it were possible to measure their behaviors along a *normal* distribution they might be expected to fall beyond 2 standard deviations from the mean.

At either extreme of the scale outlined below, an individual is likely to have problems. Individuals located at the extreme left side of the scale locate the source of their problems in life within themselves. These are not people who know healthy guilt. Their guilt tends to be excessive and misappropriated. This excessive guilt can be erosive.

Healthy guilt can be distinguished from *neurotic* guilt by several features. As described below:

Healthy Guilt	vs	**Neurotic Guilt**
Arises from an act		Not easily associated with an act.
Can be remedied or amended		No path to making things right
Remains confined to the wrong act(s)		Extends itself beyond the wrong act
Yields better insight and living		No avenue of escape, doomed to be repeated

The scale titled *Neurotic vs Obnoxious* highlights the polarity between blaming oneself too much and blaming others too much.

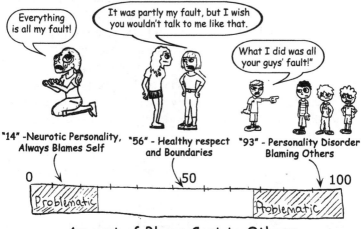

Neurotic vs. Obnoxious: "How much BLAME do you cast?"

Amount of Blame Cast to Others

On the left end of the spectrum, the *neurotic* individual blames themselves too much and too often for things that they cannot address. This person lives in a state of perpetual anxiety that their

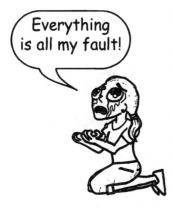

blameworthiness will be revealed. Around every bend in life is some mishap or misfortune that is surely their fault. Their ability to fault themselves knows no bounds. At times, they will blame themselves for something to which they could not even have been a party. If asked to recite the charges against them (and frequently when not asked) they do so with ease. Many self-accusations or self-reproaches are entirely fabricated. Woody Allen has made a career of portraying this sort of *neurotic* characters in comical ways. His characters did not miss an opportunity to call attention to their *neurotic* guilt and pervasive *anxiety*. While people at the extreme left end of the spectrum can prove frustrating and exhausting to their families and to clinicians, they often get along with others well enough. Although the *neurotic* blames himself, at least he also endures the suffering that results. This is in contrast to the personality disordered individual who not only blames others, but also causes others to suffer with them. Medication may provide symptom relief, but often only limited relief. Nonetheless, when symptoms are extreme and persistent, patients at the *neurotic* end of the spectrum are likely to receive antidepressants, antianxiety agents, and sleeping medication to alleviate symptoms. Psychotherapy often yields more lasting results.

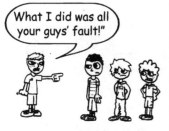

On the other end of the spectrum, the right side of the cartoon, is a figure depicting the personality-disordered domain. This person sees no fault in himself or herself, but sees endless fault in everyone else. Contrary to the New Testament teaching, these people see the spec in the other person's eye while entirely missing the log in their own. The particular personality disorder chosen for the illustration was a young man with narcissistic personality disorder whose hubris leaves him feeling entitled to blame everyone but himself. Certain personality disorders (borderline and narcissistic) tend to provoke very strong emotion in others, including clinicians. Clinicians must guard against acting in accord with the very intense, distorted projections from the patient (countertransference). This is sometimes terribly difficult to avoid since patients sometimes use very crafty, covert means to "stir things up". Medications are rarely helpful; however, when symptoms of distressing emotions become severe enough, antidepressants, antianxiety agents, mood stabilizing agents, antipsychotic agents, and sleeping agents are frequently employed. Though psychotherapy can be very helpful in some instances, some individuals with borderline and narcissistic personality disorders have difficulty tolerating the intensity of a one-on-one, dyadic psychotherapy relationship. Such individuals may find *Dialectical Behavior Therapy* helpful since this highly structured approach tends to diffuse some of the intensity of individual therapy while providing tools for regulating affect and improving interpersonal effectiveness. A perennial problem in treating any of the personality disorders is their unyielding tendency to locate their difficulties outside themselves. Other people often recognize the need for treatment long before they do. Clinicians should remain alert for signs that the patient is distorting the relationship, making the clinician the blameworthy party for their own behavior. After all, this feature is so entrenched that it does not yield to life experience.

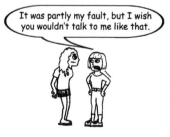

It was partly my fault, but I wish you wouldn't talk to me like that.

In the middle region a person demonstrates the ability to accept responsibility for their actions without unnecessary or exaggerated self-reproach. At the same time, a person in the middle is able to discern that others sometimes share in responsibility and can be held accountable when something goes awry. In the middle of the scale a person demonstrates fluidity and flexibility in the way they adapt to challenges and problems life presents. Holding the center of this *Spectrum* is particularly difficult and too often the extremes are reserved for the ones closest to us.

CONCLUSION

Personality consists of those traits that are stable and persist over time. Personality Disorders are defined by persistent traits that are *maladaptive*. The central idea presented in this chapter is that *personality disorders* locate the cause of their problems outside themselves. This one trait makes it difficult to adapt to life's demands since a person's efforts are directed almost exclusively to fixing others and not themselves. The *neurotic* end of the spectrum revolves around blaming oneself. Here the impediment to change is the grip of unfounded self-reproach that tends to defeat the neurotic individual.

Life demands of each of us a willingness to accept our role in matters that go wrong without yielding to an exaggerated degree of self-reproach or self-criticism. When that balance is struck, a person learns from their mistakes, they cultivate a forgiving attitude toward themselves and others, and they develop the capacity to deal with the role that others play in their misfortunes.

SECTION III

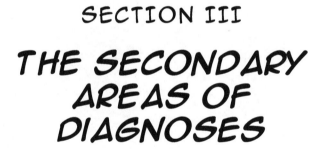

THE SECONDARY
AREAS OF
DIAGNOSES

THE SPECIALTY AREAS (TRAUMA, NEURODEVELOPMENTAL, NEUROCOGNITIVE, BEHAVIORAL, DISSOCIATIVE, SOMATIC, EATING, ELIMINATION, SLEEP, SEXUAL, GENDER, PARAPHILIA)

The remaining sections of DSM-5 are covered in this section titled "The Specialty Areas." These disorders do not lend themselves to inclusion as *Primary Spectrums, as* they lack the quality of universality. To some extent, everyone can be understood to have features associated with the *8 Primary Spectrums of Mental Illness.* Although the Specialty Areas perhaps can also be conceptualized along a dichotomous spectrum, for the sake of simplicity and clarity they are not elucidated as part of the *Primary Spectrums of Mental Illness* developed in this book.

TRAUMA- AND STRESSOR-RELATED DISORDERS

Trauma- and Stressor-Related Disorders are very common. In a telephone interview study by Resnick, "Lifetime exposure to any type of traumatic event was 69%, whereas exposure to crimes that included sexual or aggravated assault or homicide of a close relative or friend occurred among 36%. Overall sample prevalence of PTSD was 12.3% lifetime and 4.6% within the past 6 months."[24] Individuals differ with regard to the effects they suffer when confronting a trauma or stress.

By segregating *Trauma- and Stressor-Related Disorders* DSM-5 gives clear emphasis to "persistent negative alterations in mood and cognition". *Trauma- and Stressor-Related Disorders* include *Post Traumatic Stress Disorder (PTSD), Acute Stress Disorder, Adjustment Disorders,* and *Reactive Attachment Disorder.* PTSD can now be applied to individuals who experience a trauma indirectly. Two subtypes are recognized, PreSchool Subtype (<6 y.o.) and Dissociative Subtype. In DSM-5 *Adjustment Disorders* are recognized to be related to a stress and therefore no longer does *Adjustment Disorder* appear under the section of mood disorders.

NEURODEVELOPMENTAL DISORDERS

The Neurodevelopmental Disorders include diagnoses that are typically recognized in childhood: *Autism Spectrum Disorder (ASD), Attention Deficit Hyperactivity Disorder (ADHD), Communication Disorder, Specific Learning Disorder, and Motor Disorders.*

ADHD is virtually unchanged. *Reading Disorder, Mathematics Disorder,* and *Disorder of Written Expression* have all been combined into *Specific Learning Disorder.*

The diagnosis of *Mental Retardation* has been replaced by *Intellectual Developmental Disorder.* This disorder is now assessed more by adaptive functioning and less by absolute IQ score.

NEUROCOGNITIVE DISORDERS

DSM-IV's diagnosis of *Dementia* has seen a substantial shift in the new schema. The term *Dementia* has been replaced with *Neurocognitive Disorder.* A spectrum of functioning is now recognized by distinguishing *Mild Neurocognitive Disorders* from *Major Neurocognitive Disorders.* The *Neurocognitive Disorders* include a long list of subtypes that specify the particular cause of the disorder. Subtypes include: *Alzheimer's, Vascular, Substance Induced, Traumatic Brain Injury, HIV Infection, Parkinson's Disease, Lewy Bodies, Prion Disease,* and *Huntington's Disease.*

DISRUPTIVE, IMPULSE-CONTROL, AND CONDUCT DISORDERS

Listed under this heading are *Oppositional Defiant Disorder, Conduct Disorder, Antisocial Personality Disorder, Pyromania, Kleptomania.*

DISSOCIATIVE DISORDERS

Dissociative Disorders comprises a separate category in DSM-5, and *Depersonalization Disorder* has been changed to *Depersonalization/Derealization Disorder.* Dissociative Fugue is noted as a *Specifier* in DSM-5.

SOMATIC DISORDERS

 Somatic Symptom Disorder is a new construct in DSM-5. This disorder can easily be conceived as existing along a *spectrum* ranging from the previously recognized diagnosis of Hypochondriasis to Somatiztion Disorder. With DSM-5, Somatization Disorder, Hypochondriasis, Pain Disorder, and Undifferentiated Somatoform Disorder have all been eliminated and replaced by the *Somatic Symptom Disorder Diagnosis.* The centerpiece of this disorder involves the extent to which the patient experiences distressing feelings, thoughts, or behaviors out of proportion to what might be expected from a condition. This disorder shifts the focus away from "unexplained medical symptoms". Clinicians may have experienced patients who were enraged by the implication that they had "made up" their symptoms. The introduction of *Somatic Symptom Disorder* circumvents this issue.

FEEDING AND EATING DISORDERS

 DSM-5 adds a new category within the text, *Feeding and Eating Disorders*. It encompasses eating disorders typically found in children, adolescents, and adults. *Pica* and *Rumination Disorder* can now be diagnosed at any age.

 Avoidant/Restrictive Food Intake Disorder, a newly created diagnosis, is primarily intended to be used for children with extreme food preferences leading to substantial psychological or nutritional problems.

Women no longer must have had amenorrhea to meet criteria for *Anorexia Nervosa*.

The required frequency of purging behavior in *Bulimia Nervosa* changes from twice per week to once per week.

 Binge – Eating Disorder is for individuals who have weekly loss of control resulting in overeating leading to significant distress.

SLEEP DISORDERS

Sleep disorders have been recategorized to show a more fluid spectrum between medical and psychological issues. Primary insomnia has been renamed *Insomnia Disorder*. *Breathing-Related Sleep Disorders* now include *Obstructive Sleep Apnea, Central Sleep Apnea*, and a new category called *Sleep-Related Hypoventilation*.

 Rapid Eye Movement Sleep Behavior Disorder and *Restless Leg Syndrome* are newly created diagnoses.

GENDER DYSPHORIA

The creation of the new diagnosis in DSM-5, *Gender Dysphoria*, represents an acknowledgment of the substantial psychological, political, and societal changes that have taken place during the past 20 years since the release of DSM-IV. The removal of the term *identity disorder* and its replacement with a concept of *gender incongruence* that has the potential to produce *dysphoria* and problems *adapting* may have lasting implications. To those in the LGBTQ (lesbian, gay, bisexual, transgendered, queer) community this new conceptualization gives more appropriate emphasis to the individuals' distress and dysphoria. By disengaging *Gender Dysphoria* from the category of sexual dysfunctions and paraphilias where DSM-IV placed it, the DSM-5 may be expected to decrease stigmatization.

SEXUAL DYSFUNCTIONS

The Sexual Dysfunctions section has been reorganized in DSM-5. *Vaginismus* and *Dyspareunia* have been removed from the manual and replaced with *Genito–Pelvic Pain/Penetration Disorder*. Furthermore, the diagnosis of *Sexual Aversion Disorder* has been removed due to a lack of research evidence to support its inclusion.

PARAPHILIC DISORDERS

This category is virtually unchanged.

SECTION IV

CONCLUSIONS

CHAPTER 14

THE HARMONY OF THE LOTUS FLOWER

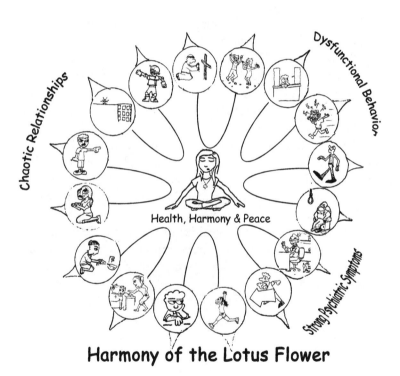

Health, Harmony & Peace

Harmony of the Lotus Flower

This illustration is a mandala giving both a summary of our schema as well as a vision of how optimal functioning might look. It includes the *8 Primary Psychiatric Spectrums* radiating from the center of the Lotus flower. The 8 spectrums are paired and joined together by a parabola whose apex comes together with the other pairs at the center of the flower. This spot at the apex of the parabola is the middle range of each of the 8 spectrums. This is the "sweet spot" that we try to attain for each continuum. On the periphery of the flower are the extreme ends of each spectrum. As there are 8 primary psychiatric spectrums there are 16 poles altogether, 2 for each spectrum. When we optimize each of the 8 primary spectrums, and find ourselves mostly in the center of the Lotus, we achieve balance, flexibility, and adaptability. We represent this by the person peacefully meditating in the Lotus flower's central space. Such states of balance may be elusive but it is a personal call, a challenge.

This "center point" of the image is referred to by many names. It can be described as "being present in the moment," "living in the now," "staying aware," "being in flow," or "being in the zone." Some may experience it as a spiritual space of feeling closer to God or an intense clarity. As clinicians, part of our job is to assist clients in their struggles to pull toward the center of each of the 8 spectrums and remain in that optimal zone.

The ultimate goal may be a state of transcendence of the apparent dialectical splits present in each spectrum. This involves holding the opposite ends of each spectrum in tension and embracing something new that seeks to emerge. The new state is more than a 50/50 balance between the opposite poles; it is something entirely different that preserves the qualities of the initial elements. We recognize when transcendent figures appear such as Martin Luther King Jr., Mahatma Gandhi, Jesus, and others. Here lies our ultimate calling.

CHAPTER 15

CARL JUNG AND HIS RELATIONSHIP TO DSM-5

The simplification of DSM-5 presented in this book fits well with most schools of psychology. It is equally at home with Cognitive Behavioral Therapy, Object Relations, Self-Psychology, and other theoretical systems. Like the DSM, this book attempts to be "atheoretical," meaning it is much more descriptive and less representative of any particular theoretical perspective.

However, there is a decidedly Jungian aspect to the way this book presents the concept of *Spectrums of Illnesses*.

Carl Jung, a Swiss born psychiatrist and contemporary of Sigmund Freud was an original thinker and courageous explorer of the psyche. He and Freud parted ways in 1913 and Jung went on to found the school of Analytical Psychology that he wanted to name Complex Psychology. Some of the notable ideas introduced by Jung and his followers include archetypes, collective unconscious, complexes, persona, shadow, introversion, extroversion, and individuation.

Part of Jung's concept of the psyche includes a *transcendence of opposites*. Jung writes "The confrontation of the two positions generates a tension charged with energy and creates a living, third thing—not a logical stillbirth in accordance with the principle *tertium non datur* but a movement out of the suspension between opposites, a living birth that leads to a new level of being, a new situation. The transcendent function manifests itself as a quality of conjoined opposites." (Jung, CW 8, par. 189). Jung further writes "But if a union is to take place between opposites like spirit and matter, conscious and unconscious, bright and dark, and so on, it will happen in a third thing, which represents not a compromise but something new, just as for the alchemists the cosmic strife of the elements was composed by the stone that is no stone, by a transcendental entity that could be described only in paradoxes." (Jung, CW 14, par. 765)

Jung felt that one of the requirements of psychological growth is to learn how to hold polar opposites despite their contradictions and maintain that tension in our psyche until a transcendent third element appeared. The transcended third was not just a compromise between two opposites, but something entirely new, perhaps even revolutionary.

In our model, holding the opposites of the *8 Primary Psychiatric Spectrums* is not merely an attempt to stay in some sort of homeostatic balance. Ideally, it fosters the transcendence of opposites wherein a new state of consciousness and being emerges. This is quite similar to Jung's description of the "transcendent function". It is the state of "living in the moment" and offers complete freedom to be responsive to each moment. We are called to live as something bigger than the sum of our balanced parts. We are ultimately a transcendent spiritual being listening to a higher call. That is the ultimate *Harmony of the Lotus Flower.*

ON ICD-10 AND THE DSM-5

The International Classification of Disease (ICD-10) differs substantially from the DSM-5. DSM-5 was developed by the American Psychiatric Association in order to better define clinical practice within mental health; it strives for a common diagnostic language. DSM-5's principal focus is improved clinical care through more accurate and widely accepted diagnoses. Practically, it is also a means by which insurance claims are coded and submitted for the purpose of reimbursement. ICD-10 on the other hand, is an international classification system developed by the World Health Organization (WHO) to provide uniform diagnoses in all fields of medicine worldwide. The objective is grounded in the tact that ICD-9 is outdated and no longer workable for treatment, diagnosis, and reimbursement. More specific data provided by ICD-10 is expected to provide better information for identifying diagnosis, public health trends, epidemics, and even bio-terrorism events. There is also a hope that precision in coding will result in fewer rejected claims, improved quality of care, and more useful benchmarks for data gathering and analysis.

The deadline for adoption of ICD-10 in the United States is set for October 1, 2015. Despite repeated delays, or perhaps because of such delays, many clinicians remain skeptical of this deadline. Prior deadlines for adoption of ICD-10 in the US have included 2011, 2012, 2013, and 2014. ICD 10's predecessor has been in use in the US for the past 35 years. ICD-9 has approximately 13,000 diagnostic codes; whereas, ICD-10 has a staggering 68,000 codes.

ICD-10 has substantially expanded how clinicians code their diagnoses for reimbursement. For the general practitioner and many specialties in medicine this is daunting. While ICD-9 had 3–5 digits in each code, ICD-10 has up to 7 digits per code. Many medical practitioners using ICD-10 must code each illness not only to a specific diagnosis, but also a particular etiology, severity, and body location. This greatly adds both to the length of the code and an increased number of variations.

ICD-10 is divided into 26 sections, one for each letter of the alphabet. Thus, the 26 sections begin with A, B, C, D, etc..... Each lettered section has a different area of medicine that it covers. Sections A and B cover infectious diseases; section C is oncology; section D is hematology...etc. The mental health codes are in section "F." Thus, virtually all the mental health codes begin with the letter "F." Luckily for a mental health practitioner, it is a fairly straightforward translation from the old ICD-9 codes to the newer ICD-10. This is mostly because mental health does not have different "body parts" that are affected and most mental illness has no clearly defined etiology. Thus, the majority of the old ICD-9 mental health codes have a one-to-one correlation with their newer ICD-10 counterparts.

ICD-10's "F Section" for mental illness is broken down into 10 subsections as follows:

F01-F09 Mental disorders due to clear physiological conditions

F10-F19 Mental disorders due to substance abuse

F20-F29 Schizophrenia, schizotypal, delusional, and other psychotic processes

F30-F39 Mood disorders

F40-F48 Anxiety, dissociative, stressor-related, and somatoform disorders

F50-F59 Behavioral syndromes with physical factors

F60-F69 Personality Disorder

F70-F79 Intellectual disabilities

F80-F89 Pervasive developmental disorders

F90-F98 Disorders of childhood and adolescence

F99-F99 Unspecified mental disorders

This book includes a section with the majority of DSM-5 as well as ICD-10 summarized into a few pages. This is meant to serve as a quick reference for the commonly diagnosed mental disorders. While it summarizes the diagnostic criterion, it does not have the entire set of criterion. Likewise the main ICD-10 codes used on a daily basis appear in the forward. With each common diagnosis you will see the DSM-5 code listed on the left, followed by the "F-code" for ICD-10 right after it. Reviewing these pages will give you a quick refresher of both systems.

BIBLIOGRAPHY

1. Kapur, S., A. G. Phillips, and T. R. Insel. "Why Has It Taken so Long for Biological Psychiatry to Develop Clinical Tests and What to Do about It?" *Molecular Psychiatry* 17, no. 12 (2012): 1174-179. doi:10.1038/mp.2012.105.
2. Insel, Thomas. "Director's Blog: Transforming Diagnosis." NIMH RSS. April 29, 2013. Accessed September 14, 2014. http://www.nimh.nih.gov/about/director/2013/transforming-diagnosis.shtml
3. Jung, C. G. "The Phenomenology of the Spirit in Fairytales." In *Collected Works of C.G. Jung Volume 9, Part 1: The Archetypes and the Collective Unconscious,* 397. Vol. 9. London: Routledge and Kegan Paul, 1959.
4. "And do not give the weak-minded your property, which Allah has made a means of sustenance for you, but provide for them with it and clothe them and speak to them words of appropriate kindness." "Surat An-Nisa' (The Women) - ءاسنلا ةروس." Surat An-Nisa' [4:5]. Accessed September 14, 2014. http://quran.com/4/5.
5. *Diagnostic and Statistical Manual of Mental Disorders: DSM-5.* Washington, D.C.: American Psychiatric Association, 2013. 22.
6. Spurgeon, Charles H. "The Sitting of the Refiner." Christian Classical Ethereal Library. Accessed October 19, 2014. http://www.ccel.org/ccel/spurgeon/sermons27.txt. Spurgeon was a renowned preacher who suffered from recurrences of gout and depression.
7. *Diagnostic and Statistical Manual of Mental Disorders: DSM-5.* Washington, D.C.: American Psychiatric Association, 2013. 271.
8. Angst, J. "The Bipolar Spectrum." *The British Journal of Psychiatry* 190, no. 3 (2007): 189–91. doi:10.1192/bjp.bp.106.030957.

9. Hollingworth, Leta Stetter. *Functional Periodicity; an Experimental Study of the Mental and Motor Abilities of Women during Menstruation.* New York: Teachers College, Columbia University, 1914.

10. Bell, Susan E., and Susan M. Reverby. "Vaginal Politics: Tensions and Possibilities in The Vagina Monologues." *Women's Studies International Forum* 28, no. 5 (2005): 430–44. doi:10.1016/j. wsif.2005.05.005.

11. Angst, J., A. Gamma, D. Clarke, V. Ajdacic-Gross, W. Rössler, and D. Regier. "Subjective Distress Predicts Treatment Seeking for Depression, Bipolar, Anxiety, Panic, Neurasthenia and Insomnia Severity Spectra." *Acta Psychiatrica Scandinavica* 122, no. 6 (2010): 488-98. doi:10.1111/j.1600-0447.2010.01580.x.

12. Angst, Jules. "Bipolar Disorders in DSM-5: Strengths, Problems and Perspectives." *International Journal of Bipolar Disorders* 1, no. 1 (2013): 12. doi:10.1186/2194-7511-1-12.

13. Moreno, C., G. Laje, C. Blanco, H. Jiang, A. B. Schmidt, and M. Olfson. "National Trends in the Outpatient Diagnosis and Treatment of Bipolar Disorder in Youth." *Archives of General Psychiatry* 64, no. 9 (2007): 1032-039. doi:10.1001/archpsyc.64.9.1032.

14. Saddock, Virginia A. "Anxiety Disorders." In *Kaplan & Sadock's Concise Textbook of Clinical Psychiatry*, by Benjamin Jesse Saddock. 3rd ed. Philadelphia, PA: Lippincott Williams & Wilkins, 2012.

15. Jakubietz, Michael, Rafael J. Jakubietz, Danni F. Kloss, and Joerg J. Gruenert. "Body Dysmorphic Disorder: Diagnosis and Approach." *Plastic and Reconstructive Surgery* 119, no. 6 (2007): 1924–930. doi:10.1097/01.prs.0000259205.01300.8b.

16. Gittelman, R., S. Mannuzza, R. Shenker, and N. Bonagura. "Hyperactive Boys Almost Grown Up: I. Psychiatric Status." *Archives of General Psychiatry* 42, no. 10 (1985): 937–47. doi:10.1001/ archpsyc.1985.01790330017002.

17. Mannuzza, S., R. G. Klein, N. Bonagura, P. H. Konig, and R. Shenker. "Hyperactive Boys Almost Grown Up: II. Status of Subjects Without a Mental Disorder." *Archives of General Psychiatry* 45, no. 1 (1988): 13–18. doi:10.1001/archpsyc.1988.01800250017003.

18. Mannuzza, S., R. G. Klein, P. H. Konig, and T. L. Giampino. "Hyperactive Boys Almost Grown Up: IV. Criminality and Its Relationship to Psychiatric Status." *Archives of General Psychiatry* 46, no. 12 (1989): 1073–079. doi:10.1001/archpsyc.1989.01810120015004.

19. Mannuzza, S., R. G. Klein, N. Bonagura, P. Malloy, T. L. Giampino, and K. A. Addalli. "Hyperactive Boys Almost Grown Up: V. Replication of Psychiatric Status." *Archives of General Psychiatry* 48, no. 1 (1991): 77–83. doi:10.1001/archpsyc.1991.01810250079012.

20. Group, The Mta Cooperative. "A 14-Month Randomized Clinical Trial of Treatment Strategies for Attention-Deficit/Hyperactivity Disorder." *Archives of General Psychiatry* 56, no. 12 (1999): 1073–086. doi:10.1001/archpsyc.56.12.1073.

21. Rehm, Jürgen, Colin Mathers, Svetlana Popova, Montarat Thavorncharoensap, Yot Teerawattananon, and Jayadeep Patra. "Global Burden of Disease and Injury and Economic Cost Attributable to Alcohol Use and Alcohol-use Disorders." *The Lancet* 373, no. 9682 (2009): 2223–233. doi:10.1016/S0140–6736(09)60746-7.

22. Sanjakdar, Sarah S., Pretal P. Madoon, Micahel J. Marks, Darlene H. Bruznell, Uwe Maskos, Michael McIntosh, Scott Bowers, and Imad Damaj. "Differential Roles of α6β2* and α4β2* Neuronal Nicotinic Receptors in Nicotine- and Cocaine-Conditioned Reward in Mice." *Neuropsychopharmacology*, July 18, 2014. Accessed October 3, 2014. doi:10.1038/npp.2014.177.

23. Rotter, Julian B. "Generalized Expectancies for Internal versus External Control of Reinforcement." *Psychological Monographs: General and Applied* 80, no. 1 (1966): 1–28. doi:10.1037/h0092976.

24. Resnick, Heidi S., Dean G. Kilpatrick, Bonnie S. Dansky, Benjamin E. Saunders, and Et Al. "Prevalence of Civilian Trauma and Posttraumatic Stress Disorder in a Representative National Sample of Women." *Journal of Consulting and Clinical Psychology* 61, no. 6 (1993): 984–91. doi:10.1037//0022-006X.61.6.984.

INDEX

L

Lesbian, Gay, Bisexual, Transgendered, and Queer (LGBTQ) 23
Lotus Flower 6, 95, 98

M

Major Depressive Disorder 39, 51
Mania Spectrum 27, 41
Mental health 3, 4, 7, 40, 50, 99, 100
Mental illness 4, 5, 9, 10, 15, 23, 26, 27, 28, 100
Mental Illness 5, 6, 12, 25, 26, 27, 28, 68, 71, 73, 74, 79, 87
Mental Retardation 12, 20, 88
Diagnosis of 20
Mixed features specifiers 35
Mixed Features Specifiers 16, 17
Mood disorders 35, 57, 88, 100
Mood Disorders 16. *See also* Bipolar Disorders; *See also* Bipolar Disorders
Mood disturbance 35
Multiaxial System 12
Multiaxial system of diagnoses 12
Mutual friendship 76

N

Neurocognitive Disorders 6, 21
Neurocognitive Disorders
Delirium xxiii
Major Neurocognitive Disorder xxiii

Mild Neurocognitive Disorders xxiii, 88
Neurodevelopmental Disorders 19, 73, 88
Neurodevelopmental Disorders
Attention-Deficit / Hyperactivity Disorder (ADHD) xvii
Autism Spectrum Disorder xvii, 19, 73, 88
Communication Disorders xvii
Childhood Onset Fluency Disorder xvii
Language Disorder xvii
Social (Pragmatic) Communication Disorder xvii
Speech Sound Disorder xvii
Intellectual Disability xviii
Motor Disorders xviii, 19, 88
Developmental Coordination Disorder xviii
Persistent Motor or Vocal Tic Disorder xviii
Provisional Tic Disorder xviii
Stereotypic movement Disorder xviii
Tourette's Disorder xviii
Specific Learning Disorders xviii
Neurotic 27, 81, 82, 84
Guilt 81
Vs Obnoxious 81
New sleep disorders 22

O

Obsessive Compulsive Disorder xv, 17, 63
And Related Disorders 63
Body Dysmorphic Disorder xv, 18, 59, 64, 104